THE
MODERN
KAMA
SUTRA

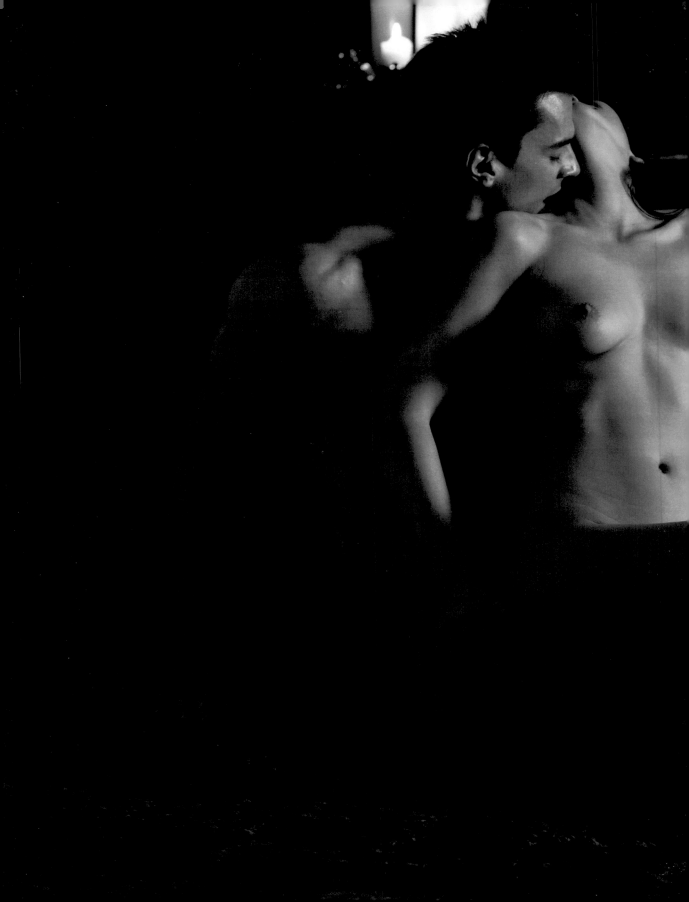

THE
MODERN
KAMA
SUTRA

ह्य

Kamini and Kirk Thomas

Photography by John Freeman

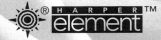

HarperElement
An Imprint of HarperCollins*Publishers*
1 London Bridge Street
London SE1 9GF

The website address is: www.thorsonselement.com

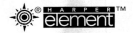

and *HarperElement* are trademarks of
HarperCollins*Publishers* Ltd

First published by HarperElement 2005
This edition 2006

14 16 18 20 19 17 15 13

© HarperElement 2005

Kamini and Kirk Thomas assert the moral right
to be identified as the authors of this work

A catalogue record of this book is
available from the British Library

ISBN 978 0 00 722976 5

Printed and bound in Hong Kong by
Printing Express Ltd

Photography by John Freeman

Art direction by XAB Design

Designed by WheelhouseCreative.co.uk

Selected photographs of Indian Statues supplied
by Nirgrantha Berghausen/ArtsErotica.com

CONTENTS

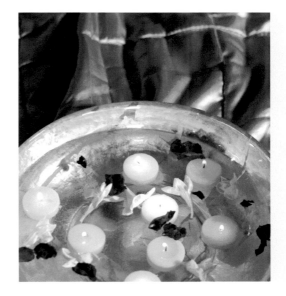

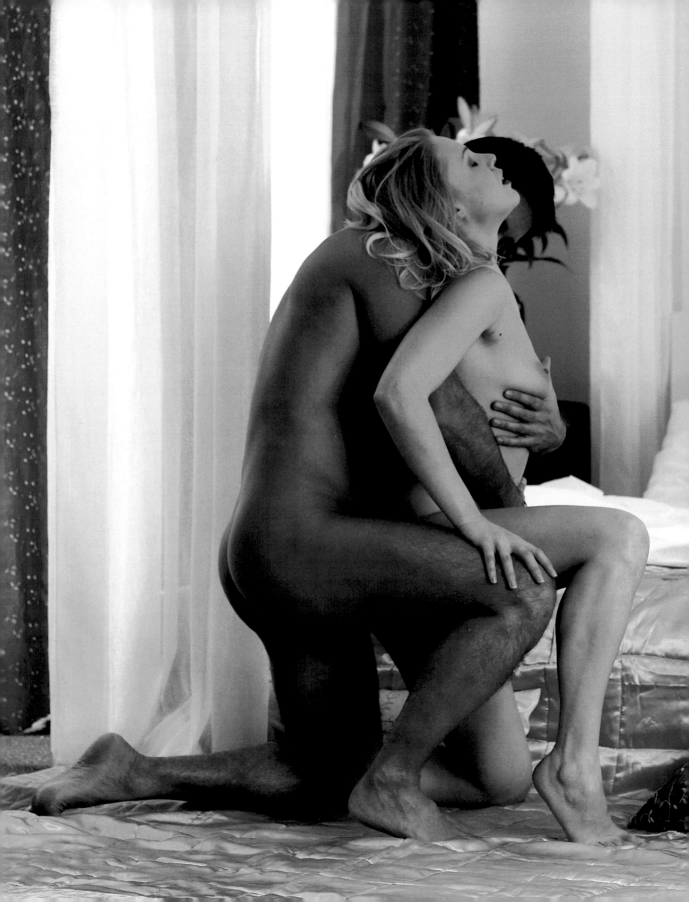

introduction

'If men and women act according to each other's
liking, their love for each other will not be lessened
even in one hundred years.'
Kama Sutra

Sex is the chemistry of love and our most primal instinct. Since the beginning of time, men and women have indulged their senses in physical union, yet attitudes towards sex have varied greatly across centuries and throughout cultures.

Many would consider the West to have more liberal views when it comes to sex, but it is actually the ancient cultures of the East that have a longstanding tradition of erotic guides or love manuals. One only needs to study the ornate sculptured façades of the medieval Hindu temples at Khajuraho and Orissa, or the intricate art depicting the romantic love between Krishna and Radha to see how the pleasures of sex were enjoyed and celebrated. These sculptures and paintings invariably have their source in the most famous treatise on sex ever composed – the *Kama Sutra*.

Ever since an elderly Indian sage named Mallinaga Vatsyayana set down a series of *sutras* or 'aphorisms' on love over two thousand years ago, the *Kama Sutra* has been a source of inspiration in the art of sensual pleasure. Little is known of Vatsyayana, about his origins, his life, or even his own loves, other than that he wrote his work whilst engaged as a religious student in the holy city of Benares. Some historians maintain that he took an oath of celibacy, though he tells us himself that, after reading the texts of ancient authors, he then followed the ways of enjoyment mentioned in them.

In studying the writings of holy men who preceded him, Vatsyayana learnt of Nandi, the white bull, who stood guard for the gods Shiva and Parvati outside their bedroom in the palace of Mount Kailash, while they made love for 10,000 years. Nandi was sworn never to speak of this, but he broke his vow and the words he uttered fell as flowers and were collected up and strung on *sutras*, or threads. These were woven into a book of 1,000 chapters. Over time, this was abbreviated to 500 chapters, then abridged to 150 and finally condensed by Vatsyayana himself into seven parts.

With scientific thoroughness and disciplined brevity, Vatsyayana describes all aspects of love and sexual relationships: from seduction and love-making to education, marriage, and conjugal life; from the ideals and accomplishments of young urban men to the life of courtesans and women of the king's harem. Even sex aids, aphrodisiacs and love potions have their place.

His text was composed 'for the benefit of the world' but he meant it as more than just an instrument to satisfy man's desires; he maintained that a person who achieved balance and harmony between the main strands of life according to Hindu scripture – virtue or religious merit (*Dharma*), worldly wealth (*Artha*) and pleasure or sensual gratification (*Kama*) – would obtain success in every undertaking and ultimately would achieve spiritual emancipation.

Though often addressed to men, the *Kama Sutra* is not only concerned with the male perspective. Vatsyayana recommended that young women should also study the work before marriage and, with the consent of their husbands, should continue to familiarize themselves with its arts thereafter because 'even the bare knowledge of them gives attractiveness to a woman'.

Divine Love

In Hindu thought, sex is not only considered natural and necessary but almost sacred, mimicking in human form the creation of the world. Hindus believe that the union of *purusha* (substance) and *praktiri* (energy) is necessary for life and is symbolised by the coming together of the great Hindu god Shiva with the divine force of Shakti, the mother goddess. Temples

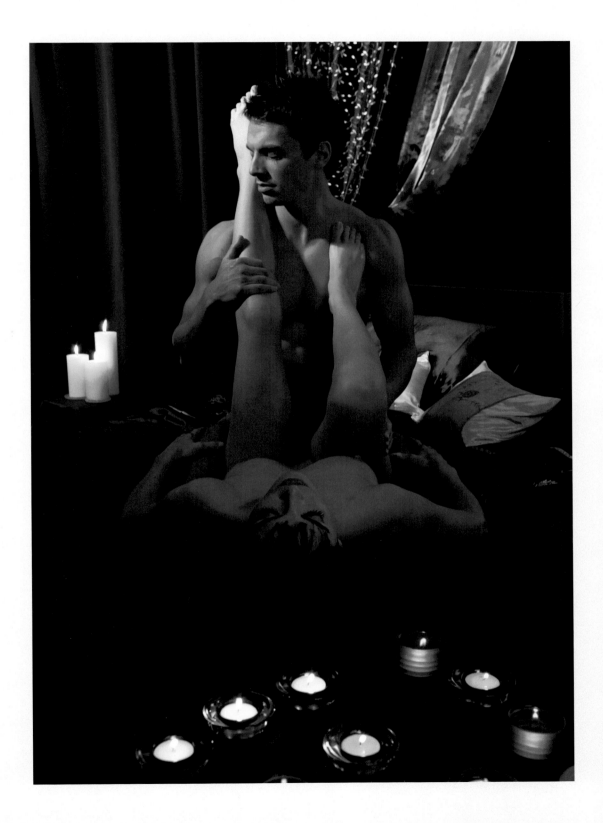

throughout India contain representations of Shiva in the form of a *lingam* (penis), whilst Shakti's symbol is the *yoni* (vagina).

This belief that men, like gods, must harness women's life-giving energy informs the writing of the *Kama Sutra*. Vatsyayana's views on the approach to a woman seem enlightened for their time: 'women, being of a tender nature, want tender beginnings,' he muses; 'the man should therefore approach the girl according to her liking, and should make use of those devices by which he may be able to establish himself more and more into her confidence.' Vatsyayana insists that the art of love is not designed to satisfy the desires of man alone; the

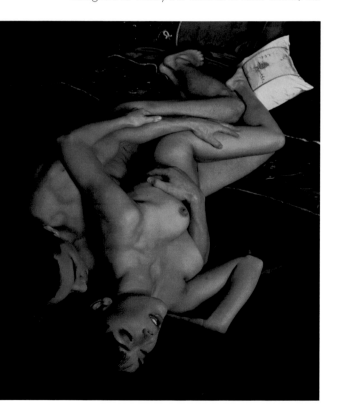

woman, too must experience the optimum delights that sensual pleasure affords, and preferably before the man has satisfied himself. Furthermore Vatsyayana maintained that, contrary to the prevailing wisdom of the time, women did indeed experience orgasm!

Citizens, Kings & Courtesans

It is thought that the *Kama Sutra* was written around the 4th century A.D., at a time of economic prosperity, when the great cities of India were flourishing and men and women of the middle and upper classes were highly educated and literate. The *Kama Sutra* certainly paints a vivid picture of a life of luxury where the *nagarika*, or city-dweller, had considerable wealth and leisure time to enjoy the pursuits and customs prevalent at the time: picnics and trips to the park to watch cock fights or to bathe, festivals honouring the gods, drinking parties, gambling, dancing, singing, reciting poetry and moonlit walks.

The wives of the king, confined in their royal harem, would resort to ingenious methods to satisfy their sexual desires if their husbands were occupied elsewhere. It was a time when courtesans were rich and cultivated and enjoyed a powerful position in society, even commanding a certain respect.

Completely lacking in prudishness, members of ancient Indian society worshipped their gods, dutifully performed their daily tasks and

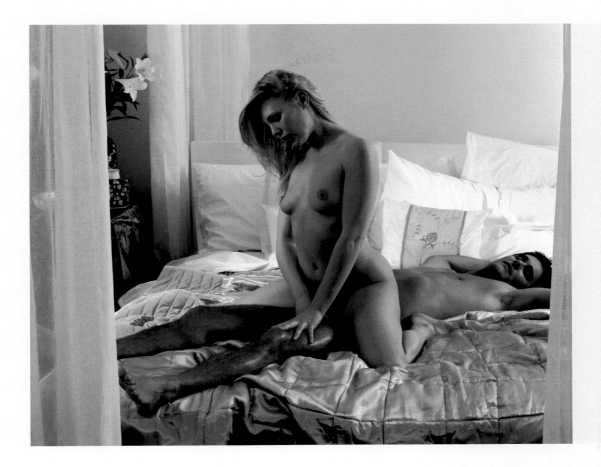

maintained the sacredness of the home, but also enjoyed life and all its pleasures to the full, believing that sexual and sensual fulfilment were as vital a part of life as final spiritual emancipation.

The *Kama Sutra* became widely read in all parts of India. Its influence permeated society, the text taken up by poets and reinterpreted and translated into song and verse. It also began to be depicted by artists and sculptors, whose artistic creations often illustrated many of the poses from the text.

The *Ananga Ranga* and the *Perfumed Garden*

The *Kama Sutra* was the first erotic manual of its kind and its importance so great that almost every subsequent sex guide to appear in India (and further afield) over the following centuries was inspired and influenced by its teaching: there was the popular *Kokashastra* by Kokkoka (containing one of the earliest mentions of the G-spot), the *Ratiratnapradipika* by Devaraja and, perhaps most prolific, the *Ananga Ranga* or 'The Hindu Art of Love'. This treatise is thought to have been composed some time during

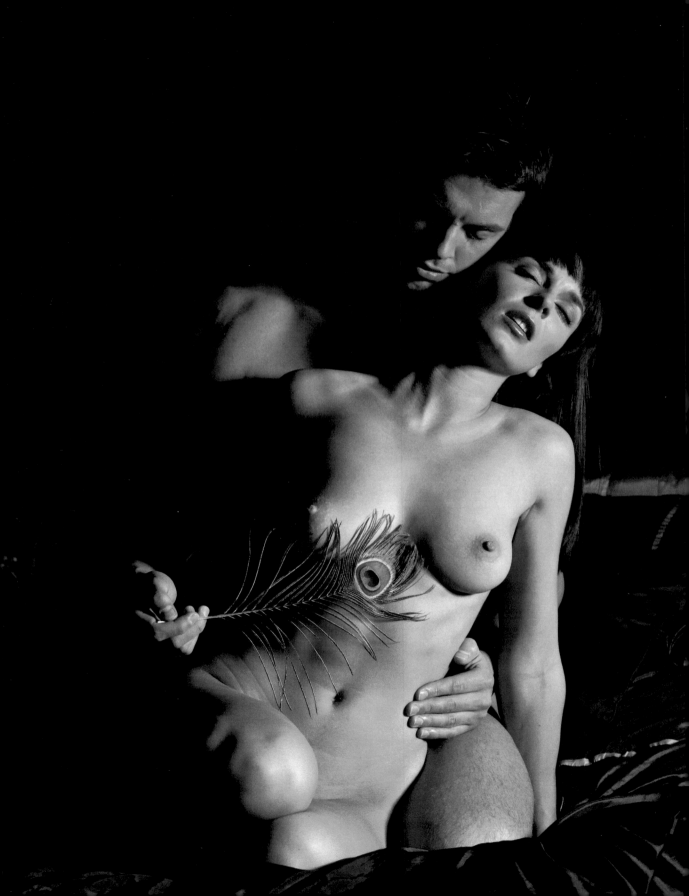

the 15th or 16th century for the amusement of Ladakhan (the son of a king) by a princely sage and arch-poet named Kalyanamalla. Society had changed since Vatsyayana's time and attitudes towards sex had become more rigid, creating boundaries between men and women. The approach of the book, therefore, is directed more towards husbands as a guide to sex within marriage, as Kalyanamalla believed that adultery was borne of monotony and the desire for varied pleasures. The *Ananga Ranga* is also a mystical guide incorporating astrology, palmistry and psychology.

The knowledge and teachings of the *Kama Sutra* slowly spread beyond India and some of its threads were gathered up by one Sheikh Nefzawi of Tunis, who set them down in his famous work the *Perfumed Garden*. The language in this love manual is frank, florid and erotic and laced with humour. For example, here is his description of the vulva:

'Such an organ is plump and outstanding in its full length; the lips are long, the opening large, the edges apart and perfectly symmetrical, and the middle prominent; it is soft, seductive, and perfect in all its details. It is, without fear of contradiction, the most agreeable and best of all. May God grant us the use of such a vulva! Amen! It is warm, narrow and dry to such a degree that one would think fire would dart from it. Its form is graceful, its odour suave; its whiteness throws the carmine centre into relief. In a word, it is perfect.'

It is interesting to know how these ancient amatory manuals came to the attention of the western world. The *Kama Sutra* of *Vatsyayana* first appeared in English in 1883, printed by the mysterious Kama Shastra Society, which was in reality none other than the Victorian adventurer and explorer Sir Richard Burton, and his friend, Forster Fitzgerald Arbuthnot, a retired Indian civil servant, who both shared a fascination for the 'Hindu erotic'.

Printed on dense paper and bound in white vellum with gold rules, the *Kama Sutra* bore the inscription 'for private circulation only'. 'It will make the British public stare,' Burton told his friend John Payne, the great Arabic scholar, on the eve of publication. Burton and Arbuthnot

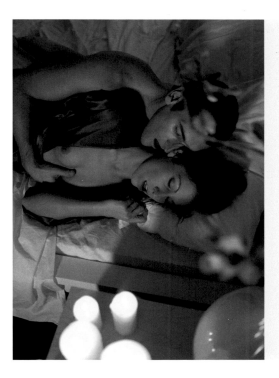

presented their work to that small selection of the public which took 'enlightened interest in studying the manners and customs of the olden east', keeping their motives vague as to how this ancient text was first brought to light. Twice reprinted between 1883 and 1885, it soon came to be regarded as a classic, which immediately altered the West's approach to Indian culture.

Burton and Arbuthnot's Kama Shastra Society followed it with a translation of the *Ananga Ranga* in 1885 (after a failed attempt to print it in the early 1870s) and the *Perfumed Garden* a year later.

The Modern Kama Sutra

This book draws principally on the ancient teachings of the *Kama Sutra*, and to a lesser extent on those of its successors. *The Modern Kama Sutra* also touches on the principles of Tantra and Yoga as well as other Eastern beliefs and practices.

Much can still be learnt from the wisdom of Vatsyayana on the themes of love, seduction and sex for modern lovers: the importance of stimulating all of the senses without becoming blinded by passion; how to be in harmony with the desires and preferences of your partner; how to create the right mood and environment to

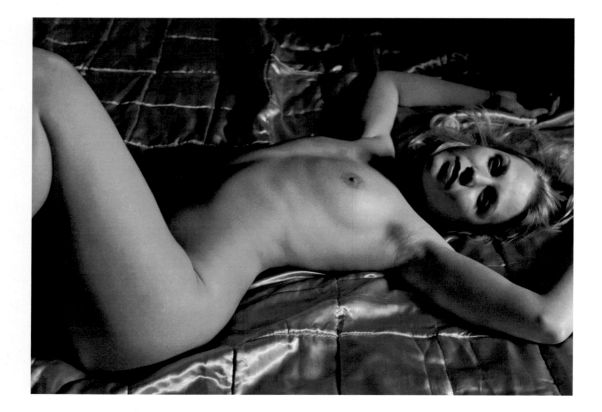

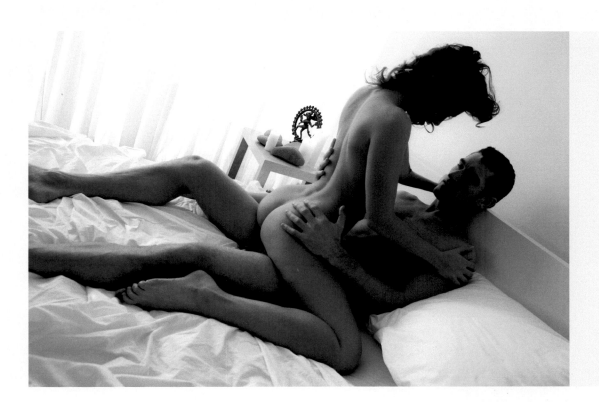

encourage feelings of intimacy and warmth; the importance of taking time to seduce your lover; and how to introduce variety into your sex life by experimenting with different positions and different styles. Above all, the *Kama Sutra* shows how best to nurture a loving, fulfilling monogamous relationship for years to come.

The sexual positions included here are drawn from all the main texts and are meant merely as a guide. The positions can be used as a series of sequences, but you do not have to follow these unswervingly; you may only want to use one at a time or try a variety in one session. There are no hard and fast rules but to help you decide there are difficulty ratings from 1–4

(1 being the easiest) and ratings by type: soft, deep, gentle, intense, slow, fast. Whatever your preferences, you can find your own favourites from the great variety of positions illustrated in the book. As Vatsyayana himself states, 'the various modes of enjoyment are not for all times or for all persons'; the idea is to experiment and create your own unique language of love.

A fully satisfying sex life requires practice and understanding. By casting off your inhibitions and opening your mind to new experiences, by paying attention to the needs and desires of your lover whilst expressing your own, you will undoubtedly reach new ecstatic heights in your sexual encounters.

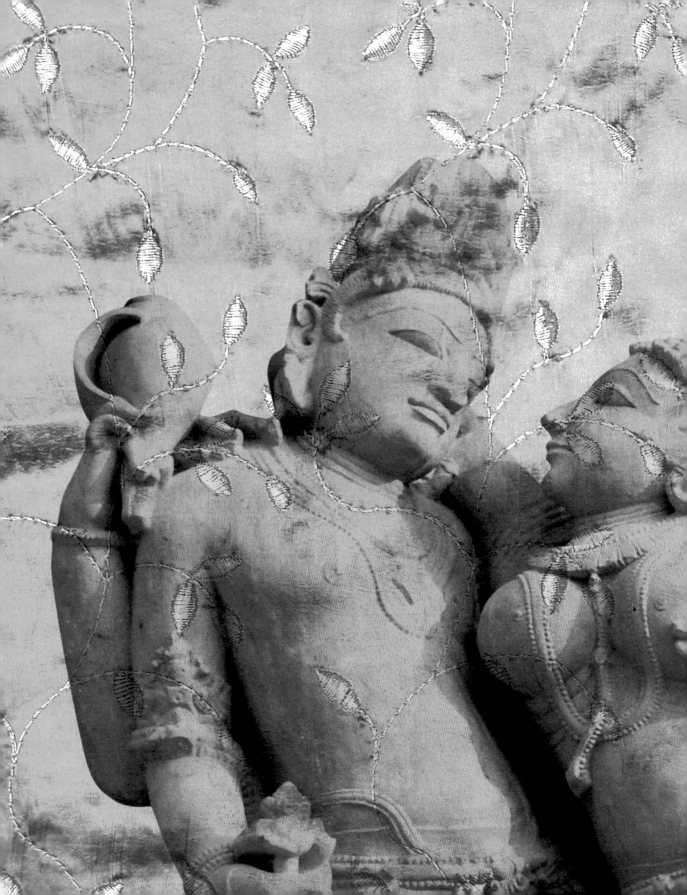

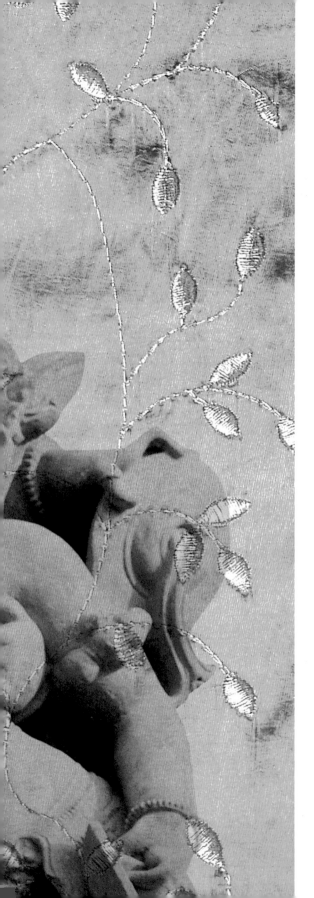

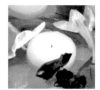

SEDUCTION

mood

body

senses

foreplay

oral sex

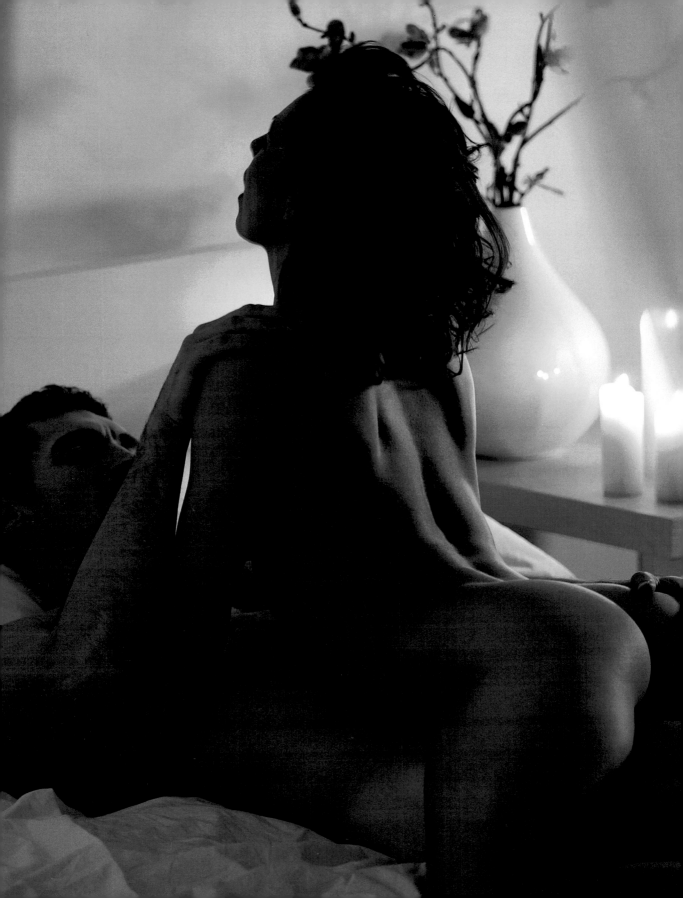

mood

'In the pleasure-room, decorated with flowers, and fragrant with perfume...the citizen should receive the woman, who will come bathed and dressed, and will invite her to take refreshment and to drink freely. He should then seat her on his left side, and holding her hair, and touching also the end and knot of her garment, he should gently embrace her with his right arm. They should then carry on an amusing conversation on various subjects, and may also talk suggestively of things which would be considered as coarse, or not to be mentioned generally in society. They may then sing, either with or without gesticulations, and play on musical instruments, talk about the arts, and persuade each other to drink...Such is the beginning of sexual union.'

Kama Sutra

Getting in the Mood

'The lovers may also sit on the terrace of the palace or house and enjoy the moonlight, and carry on an agreeable conversation. At this time, too, while the woman lies in his lap, with her face towards the moon, the citizen should show her the different planets, the morning star, the polar star, and the seven rishis, or Great Bear.'

Kama Sutra

Seduction is the temptation of our sensual desires and is an essential part of lovemaking. Drawing your lover away from the everyday concerns of life into a world of eroticism and sensuality will heighten their desire and arousal, and their experience of sex will be even more intense and pleasurable.

Initially, after a busy day, it is important to focus on your partner and share your thoughts. This will help you unwind and synchronize with each other, whether your seduction is designed to lead to the excitement of quick passionate sex or the slow-burning intensity of gradual lovemaking.

Put on calming music and turn down the lighting. Tell each other how you feel and what you'd like to do. Be explicit or merely suggestive, whatever your fancy.

Surprising each other with gifts can add to your seduction. As well as greeting one another with flowers, perfume, chocolates or wine, you could be more obvious with lingerie or sex aids or greet your partner naked at the door.

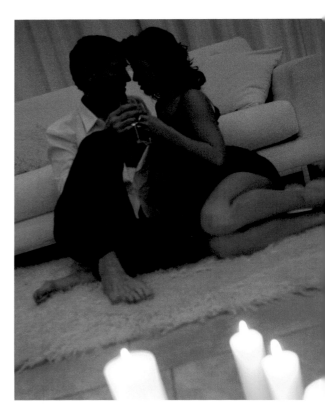

Lighting candles and a log fire if you have one will immediately soften the setting, and the scent of essential oils and incense sticks will help to stimulate your senses. Why not scatter rose petals around the bedroom or fill it with vases of flowers to create an erotic love palace. The *Kama Sutra* suggests that 'the room, balmy with rich perfumes, should contain a bed, soft, agreeable to the sight, covered with a clean white cloth, having garlands and bunches of flowers upon it'. It is important to get into the right frame of mind, and these ambient touches will help you to harmonize with your surroundings and each other.

Slowly undress one another or change into a loose robe and raunchy underwear or even dress up. Toy with one another's desires by whispering explicit comments in each other's ears or denying kisses on purpose. This loveplay and gradual arousal will allow you to attune your mind and body with your lover's, enjoying a feeling of closeness and the thrill of anticipation. You may want to vary the passion, pulling off your clothes and altering your caresses to more passionate fondling. Once you are naked, it might be hard to resist speeding things up but try to take a moment to admire each other's bodies, lingering over each part in turn.

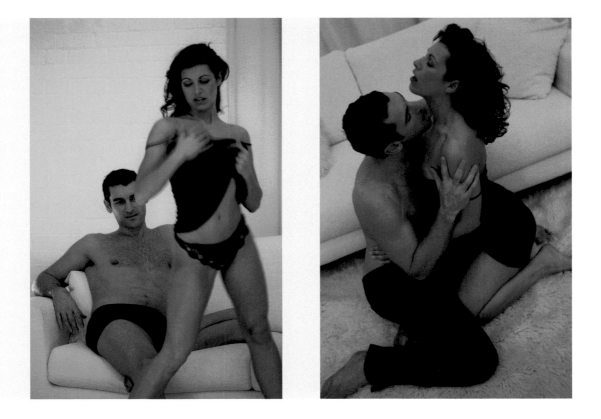

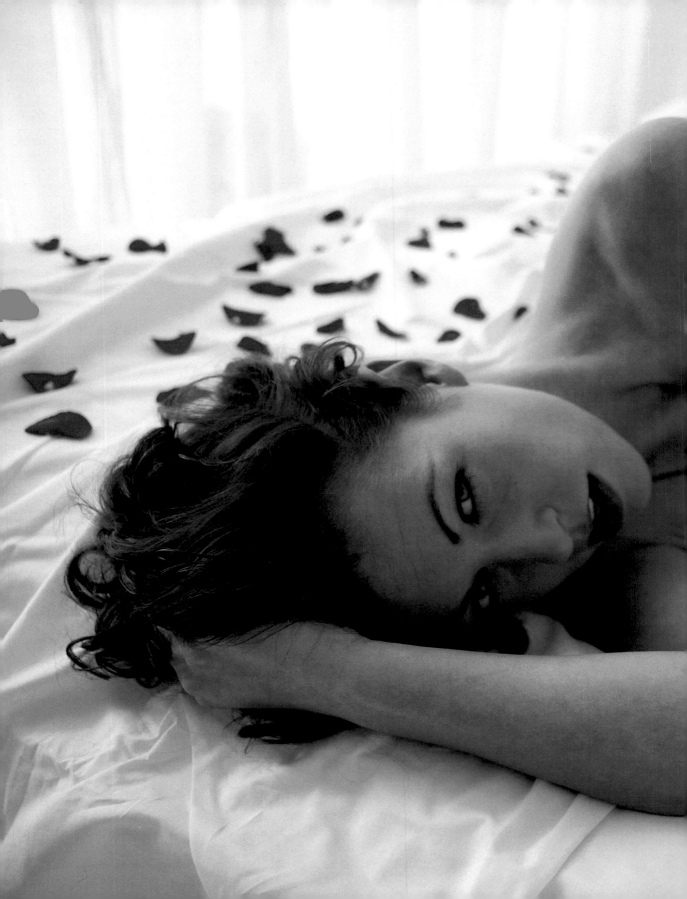

'The woman of Tirotpatna has eyes blooming like the flowers of the lake; she loves her husband fondly and her passion is enflamed by a single look; she is especially skilful in congress; she enjoys various ways and postures; and, by reason of her delicacy, she cannot endure rough or protracted embraces.'

Ananga Ranga

'The woman who before congress will touch with her left foot the lingam of her husband, and will make a practice of this, undoubtedly subdues him, and makes him her slave for life.'

Ananga Ranga

Bathing

'He should bathe daily, anoint his body with oil every other day, apply a lathering substance to his body every three days, get his head shaved every four days and the other parts of his body every five or ten days. All these things should be done without fail.'

Kama Sutra

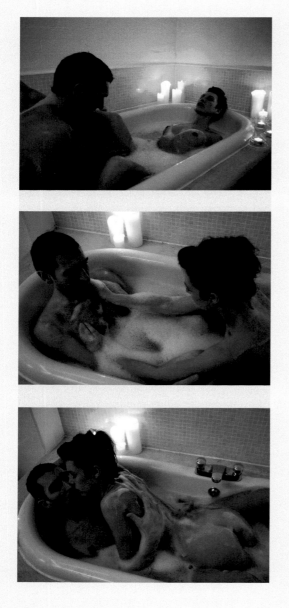

Taking a bath together is a wonderfully sensuous and intimate way to begin lovemaking. It gives you time to wind down and relax after a busy day and to explore each other's naked bodies slowly and with affection.

The bathroom can be transformed into a sensual sanctuary, where everyday distractions are washed away. Fill the bathroom with soft candlelight, add aromatherapy oils or scented bath salts to the water, and make sure the room is warm. Pour yourselves a glass of wine and luxuriate in the hot, steamy tub together.

Enjoy pampering your lover: ladle warm water all over their body, or drip cold water onto their hot skin. Focus on the moment and feel the intimacy growing between you. Talk to each other about how you feel or things you would like to do to each other.

The secret to the art of lovemaking is about taking your time. Tantalize and tease each other in the bath to build up sexual excitement. Whilst washing your lover, let your hands roam and explore, moving up towards their inner thighs and letting your fingers brush only lightly over their genitals. Try experimenting with different positions in the bath, feeling your hot wet bodies rubbing against each other. If you are so excited that you can't bear to delay the pleasure, you could masturbate each other in the bath, using the soapy water as a lubricant and letting your fingers slide back and forth.

You may prefer to take a quick shower together, which still provides an opportunity to touch and arouse each other in a warm, steamy environment. The advantage of a shower is that it is easier for bodies to be entwined and close in a standing position. The man can fondle her breasts or rub her genitals, or the woman can kneel and take his penis in her mouth.

The relaxation and gentle build-up of arousal that you have experienced in the bath or shower should be prolonged as much as possible. So, instead of hastily drying yourself off, part of your intimate ritual can include your lover enveloping you in a clean, warm towel then gently rubbing you all over. Having your most intimate parts touched with care and tenderness, without necessarily having sex, is an important part of developing a deep bond with your lover. Added to this, the rough texture of the towel against your skin can be toning, invigorating and arousing.

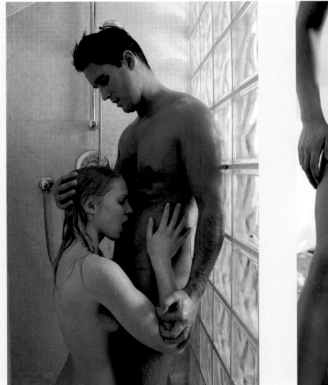
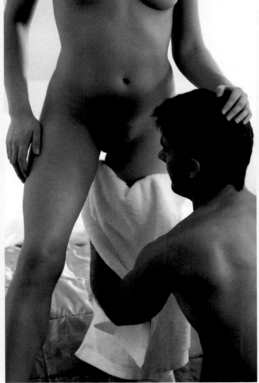

Massage

Massage has been practised for centuries in many different traditions, from Ancient Greece and Rome to Egypt and the Far East as a means of promoting healing and relaxation. Massage between partners can be a way of relaying your feelings for one another through your fingertips and of arousing each other slowly and sensually.

Massage can be applied in many different situations, whether it is a foot massage in the bath or a shoulder rub while talking. If you are planning to give your lover a full-body massage, choose somewhere comfortable like the bedroom. Lay a towel over the sheets and make sure that the room is warm.

Light a few candles and put on some calming music. A few drops of aromatherapy oils can be added to your base massage oil to help create the mood you want: juniper, patchouli, sandalwood, and ylang ylang are all powerful aphrodisiacs while jasmine, lavender and rose help to promote relaxation and feelings of well-being.

First, get into a mutually comfortable position. A good place to start is at the base of the spine, which is one of the main *chakras* (or energy points) of the body. From here, with your palms placed flat, glide your hands up the back on either side of the spine, towards the neck then across the shoulders and lightly back down

'Sitting in their own places they should eat some betel leaves and the citizen should apply with his own hand to the body of the woman some pure sandalwood ointment, or ointment of some other kind...'
Kama Sutra

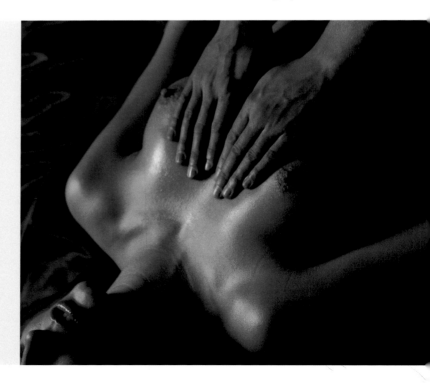

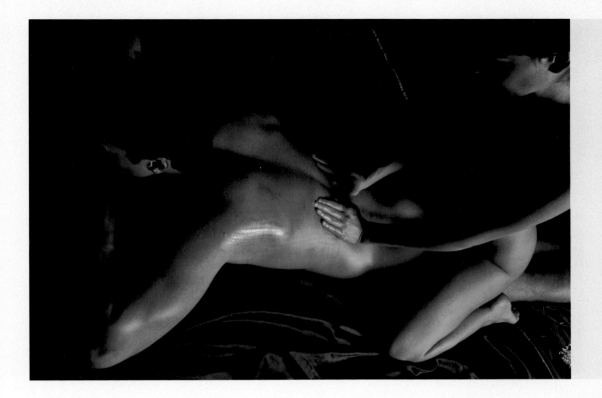

along their sides. This motion can be repeated rhythmically to build up friction and heat along the spine. Keep contact with your lover at all times and avoid any sudden or jerky movements. Ask your lover where they would like you to massage them and what kinds of stroke and pressure they prefer. If you locate a particularly knotted or tight area, use your thumbs to knead it gently to help disperse the tension.

From the back, you can work your way down the body, first kneading the muscles of the buttocks with circular motions then massaging the upper thighs, the calves, ankles and feet. Pressing on various parts of the soles of the feet can be extremely stimulating and energizing.

Turn your lover over and start by gently massaging their belly, then slide your hands upwards. The man can glide his hands around the outside of the breasts, circling them and lightly brushing the nipples with his palm as he does so.

Once your lover is fully relaxed, you can start to arouse them by using strokes that deliberately brush past their genitals. Each time you do this, linger a little longer, and when you sense that they are really turned on, you can slowly begin to masturbate them. Depending on your mood, you could bring your lover to orgasm and then lie next to them, letting them enjoy the sensation of being completely pampered, or you could continue with a warm and oily sex session.

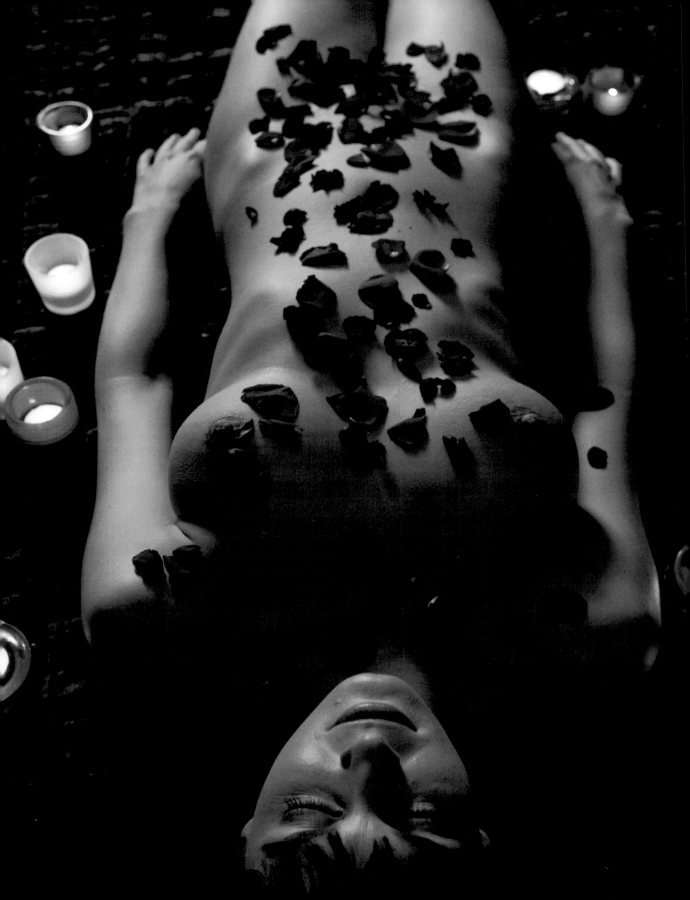

body

राा

'And here may be learned the marks whereby beauty and
good shape of body are distinguished. The maiden whose
face is soft and pleasing as the moon; whose eyes are bright
and liquid as the fawn's; whose teeth are clean as diamonds
and clear as pearls; whose neck is like a sea-shell; whose
lower lip is red as the ripe fruit of the bryony; whose hair is
black as the bee's wing; whose skin is brilliant as the flower
of the dark-blue lotus, or light as the surface of polished
gold; whose feet and hands are red, being marked with a
circle; whose voice is sweet as the Kokila-bird's – such a girl
should at once be married by the wise man.'

Ananga Ranga

The Yoni – Female Genitalia

'... it being of four kinds: that which is soft inside as the filaments of the lotus flower, this is the best; that whose surface is studded with tender flesh-knots and similar rises; that which abounds in rolls wrinkles and corrugations; that which is rough as the cow's tongue.'

Ananga Ranga

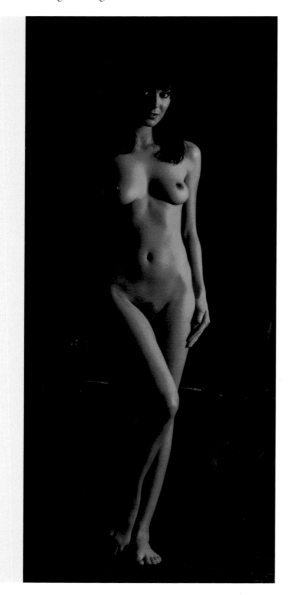

In Hindu culture, the vagina is represented by a downward triangle or trikona, being the symbol of Shakti, the divine female energy. But while the yoni was revered as the source of creation, it was also feared. The ancients believed that, like a mouth, it swallowed up and consumed the male seed. One of the many colourful names for the vagina from the *Perfumed Garden* – El âddad or The Biter – shows how the vagina was a symbol of man's unconscious fear that a woman might eat or castrate her partner during intercourse!

The female genitals are made up of several parts. The vagina is the inner part and has an average length of four inches, the G-spot located inside the first inch. The vulva is the external part of the genitals incorporating the *mons pubis* (or pubic mound), the labia, and the clitoris – one of the most sensitive points on a woman's body. The visible part, the glans, is located under the folds of skin where the labia meet at the top. This is connected to a whole network of sensitive erectile tissues extending to the pubic bone and the perineum, which swell with blood and become firm during arousal.

The Lingam – Male Genitalia

'His member should be of ample dimensions and length. Such a man ought to be broad in the chest and strong in the buttock; he should know how to regulate his ejaculation, and be quick to erect; his member should reach to the end of the canal of the female, and completely fill the same and all its parts. Such a one will be well beloved by women.'

Perfumed Garden

The penis is a universal symbol of fertility, and a potent image at the centre of many god-dominated religions. As the consort of Durga or Kali, Shiva is the erect phallus – a symbol of that which is invisible yet omnipresent – and his virile lingam is held in reverence in Hindu temples all over India, generally mounted on a circular or quadrangular receptacle called the *Avudaiyar*. In the *Kama Sutra*, men were put into three categories – the hare man, the bull man, and the horse man – according to the size of their penis, so that they would correspond with the right woman according to the depth of her vagina. This even fit made for 'equal union'.

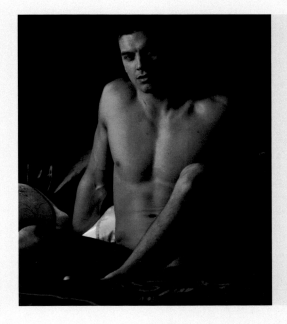

The head of the penis, the glans, is connected to the shaft by the frenulum, a thin and very sensitive stretch of skin. The shaft of the penis contains three tubes, which engorge with blood during arousal, causing the penis to swell quickly, whilst muscles at the base of the shaft contract simultaneously to stem the blood flow and help maintain erection. (The *Kama Sutra* talks of certain *Apadravyas*, or objects which are put on or around the penis in order to supplement its length or thickness.) Sperm is produced in the testicles, which are enclosed in the scrotum, which hangs below the penis. Learning to control ejaculation is essential for the enjoyment and prolonging of intercourse. As the *Kama Sutra* states, 'if a male be long-timed the female loves him the more, but if he be short-timed, she is dissatisfied'.

The Breasts

'The Yakshasatva-stri has large and fleshy breasts with a skin fair as the white champa flower; she is fond of flesh and liquor; devoid of shame and decency; passionate and irascible, and at all hours greedy for congress.'

Ananga Ranga

Every culture in the world appreciates breasts. As well as being visually pleasing, they are also powerful symbols of motherhood, nourishment and protection – the place we instinctively turn to as soon as we emerge from the womb.

For many women, the breasts are a highly sensitive erogenous zone. When aroused, the nipples harden (although it is quite common for only one nipple to be erect) and the areola becomes darker in tone. During lovemaking they provide a powerful visual and tactile stimulus for the man, but he should be aware that the breasts can be sensitive and tender and should be handled gently and not squeezed too hard.

The bosom is a warm and comforting place to nuzzle into or it can become a playground for fun and fantasy. Why not sprinkle rose petals across your lover's chest while she is lying on her back, or drip cream, yoghurt or some other delicacy over her nipples and then slowly lick it off. In the bath, cover her breasts with soapy bubbles or drip cold water on her nipples.

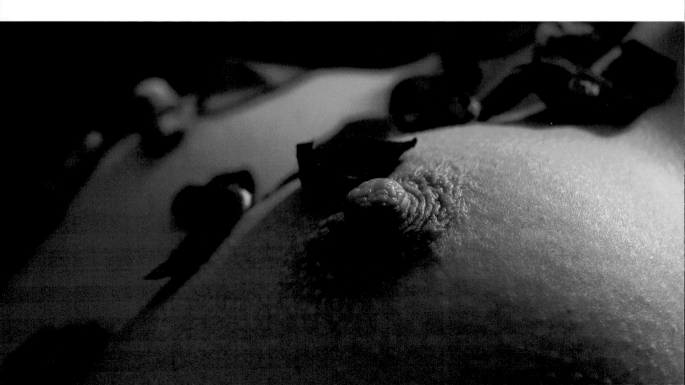

The *Kama Sutra* mentions the tradition of pressing or scratching the body with fingernails as a sign of intense passion. One of the main areas for doing this was the breast. A curved line made on the breast was called 'the tiger's nail'; indentation made with five nails was known as 'the peacock's foot'; and when they were made close to one another near the nipple, it was known as 'the jump of a hare'.

Breasts are composed mainly of fatty tissue. They have no muscles but it is possible to strengthen the ligaments that hold them and build up the pectoral muscles, which will aid posture. Try this easy exercise: with arms crossed, place your hands on your upper arms and push against them in a rhythmic pulsing action. Alternatively, you can open up your chest by raising your outstretched arms over your head.

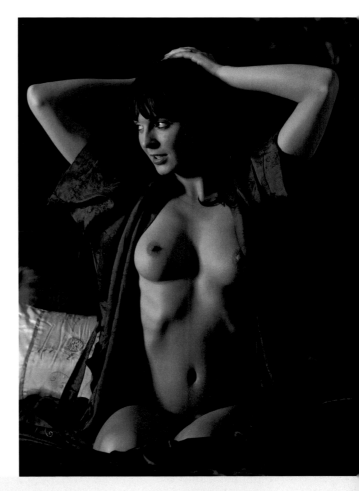

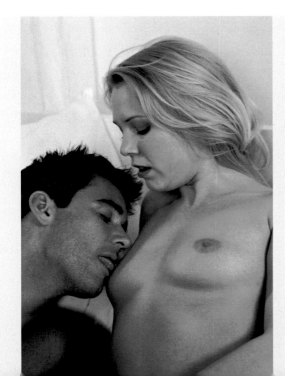

'When a woman in a lonely place bends down, as if to pick up something and pierces, as it were, a man sitting or standing with her breasts, and the man in return takes hold of them, it is called a "piercing embrace".'
Kama Sutra

The Head

'"*Kamavatansakeshagrahana*" or "*holding the crest hair of love*" is when, during the act of copulation, the husband holds with both hands his wife's hair above her ears, whilst she does the same thing to him, and both exchange frequent kisses upon the mouth.'

Ananga Ranga

Being closest to heaven, the head is deemed a sacred part of our bodies with the hair symbolizing strength and energy. Lockets of hair have long been exchanged between lovers as mementoes. And in some religions a woman's hair is kept covered, only to be revealed in private and to her husband. Hindus believed that simply by loosening her serpentine locks, the goddess Kali could unleash thunderstorms and tempests, which could only be quelled if she bound up her hair again. Similarly, Shiva's unkempt tresses were representative of wild abandon and universal sexual energy.

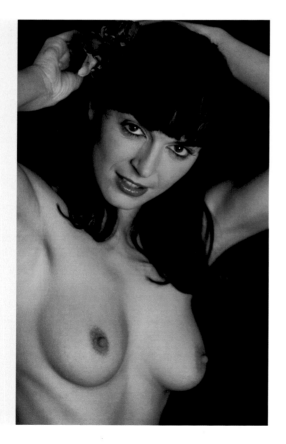

According to the *Ananga Ranga*, one of the signs that a woman is amorous, is that 'she scratches her head that notice may be drawn to it and rubs and repeatedly smooths her hair so that it may look well.' At that time most women possessed long flowing hair, which ideally was to be kept 'soft, close, thick, black and wavy'.

For centuries, hair has been used as decoration. By dressing it differently on men and women it acts as a strong gender signal, and it has often been elaborated by the use of dyes, ointments and wigs. Playing with hair can be a strong sexual signal. If you're flirting with a woman and she starts rearranging her locks you just might be in luck! The sight of a woman unbinding her hair is a real turn-on, and during sex there is nothing better than seeing your lover's hair wild and tousled.

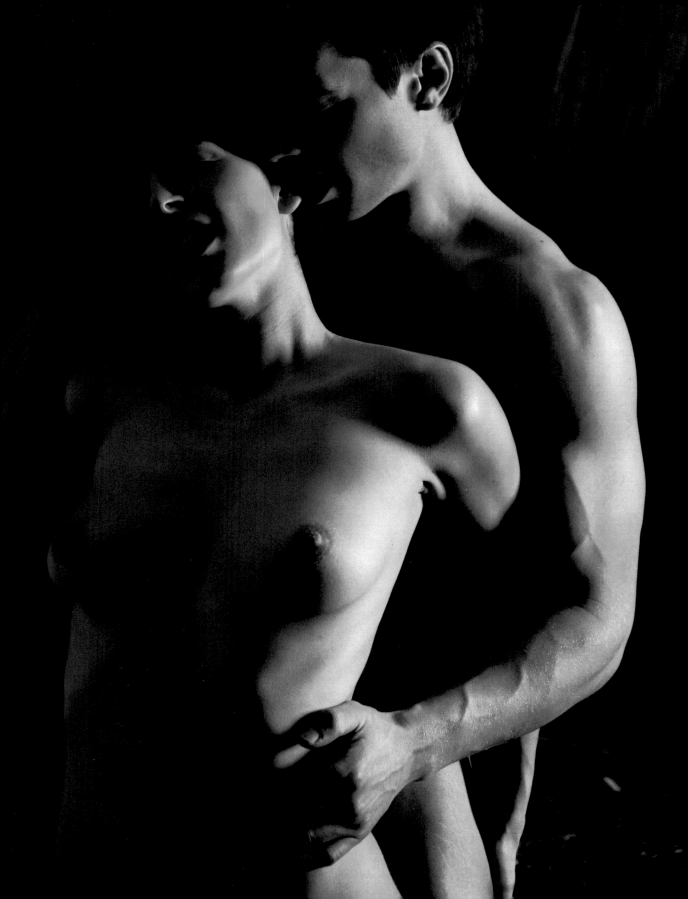

The Eyes

'The woman has eyes blooming like the flowers of the lake; she loves her husband fondly and her passion is inflamed by a single look.'

Ananga Ranga

Hindu tradition holds that all people have three eyes: two for seeing the outside world, and the third for focusing inwards towards God. This is represented by a *bindi* or dot in the centre of the forehead.

Prolonged eye contact between two people is a potent sign of love and confidence, as it allows a lover to look deep into your innermost being and leaves you open and defenceless. If you have ever had a staring match with someone, you will know just how hard it is to maintain eye contact for a long period of time. Pupil dilation is a powerful and uncontrollable indication of our attraction, and as low lighting also causes dilation this is partly why many amorous encounters take place in semi-darkness.

Flirtatious glances between lovers across a crowded room (or a boardroom table) send a thrill right through you, especially if your love is secret. By letting your eyes roam across the body of your lover and linger on their genital area, you can give powerful clues about your intentions.

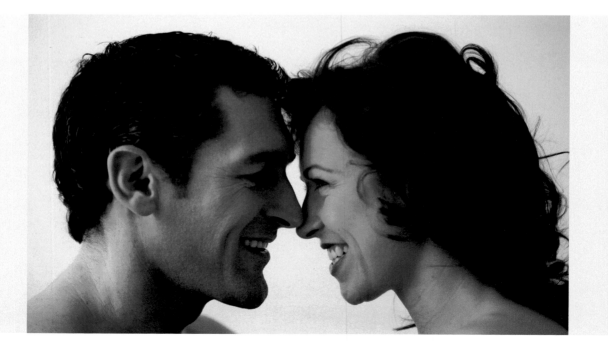

The Mouth

'She should take hold of her lover by the hair and bend his head down, and kiss his lower lip, and then, being intoxicated with love, she should shut her eyes and bite him in various places.'

Kama Sutra

The mouth is a highly erotic part of the body. It has obvious parallels with the genitals and, in ancient Hinduism, poking out the tongue was a sacred gesture, the tongue and mouth representing the linga-yoni. Even today, sticking out the tongue is a polite sign of greeting in northern India and Tibet.

In the West, pouting, slowly licking our lips or running a tongue across our teeth is highly expressive of our desires and intentions. The lips, like labia, become redder and more swollen during sexual arousal, which is undoubtedly why they have been artificially reddened with lipstick for thousands of years and, more recently, have been plumped up by collagen. The suggestive image of a woman playing with a phallic-shaped object next to her lips is often portrayed in films and magazines, and can be used during foreplay to tantalize and torment your lover. As a prelude to foreplay, eating and feeding each other tasty morsels stimulates our palate and our senses. According to the *Kama Sutra*, lovers should consume anything according to their likings as long as it is 'known to be sweet, soft, and pure.'

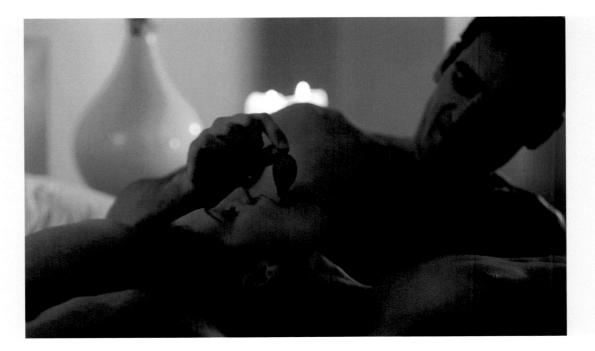

The Belly

'The woman covers up the man with her hair dishevelled, and her belly pressed with her lifted thigh, inviting the man for the union. The woman appears very beautiful in this embrace, displaying as she does the large and pleasing shape of the belly.'

Kama Sutra

In the Western world, we spend hours in the gym to get a washboard stomach, but in the East the softly rounded female form with large hips and a slightly protruding belly, or *jaghana*, is considered highly sensual and is widely depicted in erotic paintings and sculptures. The belly conceals the womb – the source of all life – and is a potent symbol of motherhood. Many women like a prolonged massage of their belly, keeping the pressure light and maintaining a consistent circular motion. If done either side of the navel, it is meant to alleviate menstrual pain, whilst just below the navel is the 'gate to the original chi', and applying slight intermittent pressure here will help shift trapped energy.

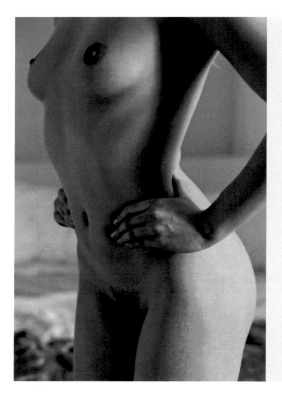

Or the woman could try belly dancing in front of her lover, adding an exotic element of fun to lovemaking. The belly roll technique is similar to the yogic practice of nauli, or churning, and is one of the principal manoeuvres in belly dancing. It is also a good way to build up muscle control. Relaxing your belly completely, place your hands against your stomach. Take in a few deep breaths and then breathe out fully. You will soon become aware of how your abdominal muscles are working. Try contracting only your upper abs, then switch to the lower ones. It will take time to develop this control, but as you do, aim to release one set of abs as you begin to contract the others. Once you have achieved the belly roll, try it in reverse so that your belly ripples down instead of up, or introduce some accompanying hip movements.

The Hands

'The man should intentionally hold her hand.'

Kama Sutra

The many hands of Indian gods like Brahma, Ganesh and Shiva symbolize diversity and omnipotence. Amongst Hindus, hand gestures are as common as words and highly significant. The most common form of greeting in India is the namaskar, made by bringing the palms together before the face or chest and bowing.

A person's hands and the way they use them to express themselves are one of the first things we notice so it is important to take care of them and make sure that they are clean and presentable. The *Kama Sutra* stresses the importance of washing and painting the hands, particularly the nails, which should be 'bright, well set, clean, entire, convex, soft and glossy in appearance'.

The extremities of our bodies contain hundreds of nerve endings – the hands alone have 17,000 tactile receptors – making them highly sensitive and very important tools in the arts of sex and seduction. With the lightest touch our hands and fingers can convey a whole world of meaning, and often far better than words, and there is no simpler expression of intimacy than interlocking fingers with your lover.

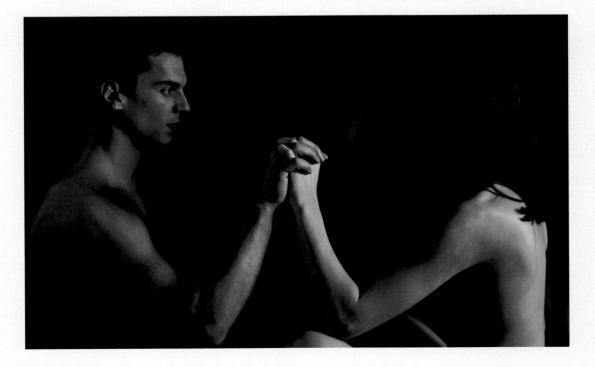

Legs & Feet

'Having placed his foot upon hers, he should slowly touch each of her toes, and press the ends of the nails; if successful in this, he should get hold of her foot with his hand and repeat the same thing. He should also press a finger of her hand between his toes when she happens to be washing his feet.'

Kama Sutra

Almost every sexual posture involves the entwining of our limbs, particularly our legs, and there are numerous depictions of awkwardly contorted limbs in most of the ancient Indian paintings and sculptures. Some of these graphic images show a prince in 'simultaneous congress' with many women of the harem, using his big toes to pleasure the clitoris of one or two consorts. If you are going to try this, make sure your nails are cut!

Indian women decorate their feet with detailed henna patterns, and adorn their toes and ankles with rings and jangling bracelets. The mere sight of a woman's legs and slender ankles is a real turn-on for many men, and the delicate female foot has long been an object of eroticism and fetish. Kissing the feet can be a sign of adoration, and toe-sucking creates wonderful sensations throughout the body.

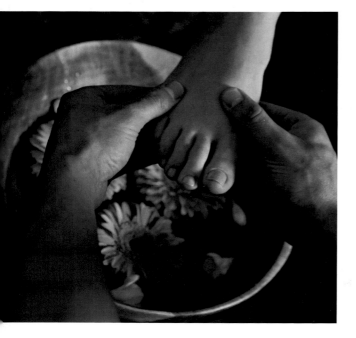

Foot Massage

After a long day, show your devotion to your lover by bathing their feet in warm water then massaging them using scented oils. There are hundreds of reflex points on the feet that correspond to all the parts of the body. By stimulating and applying pressure to these points you are stimulating the whole body, which can create powerful feelings of relaxation and well-being.

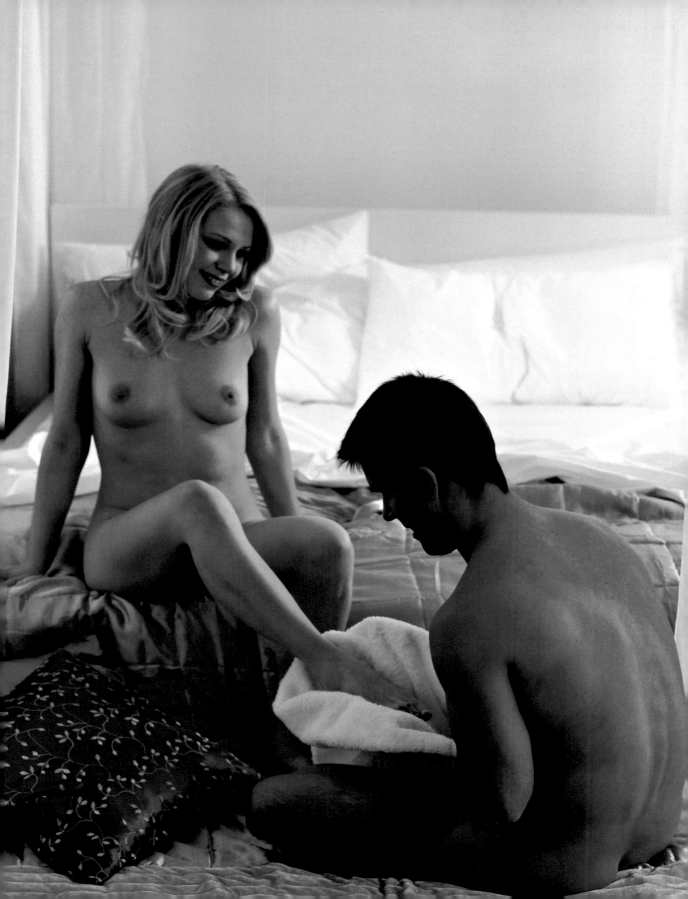

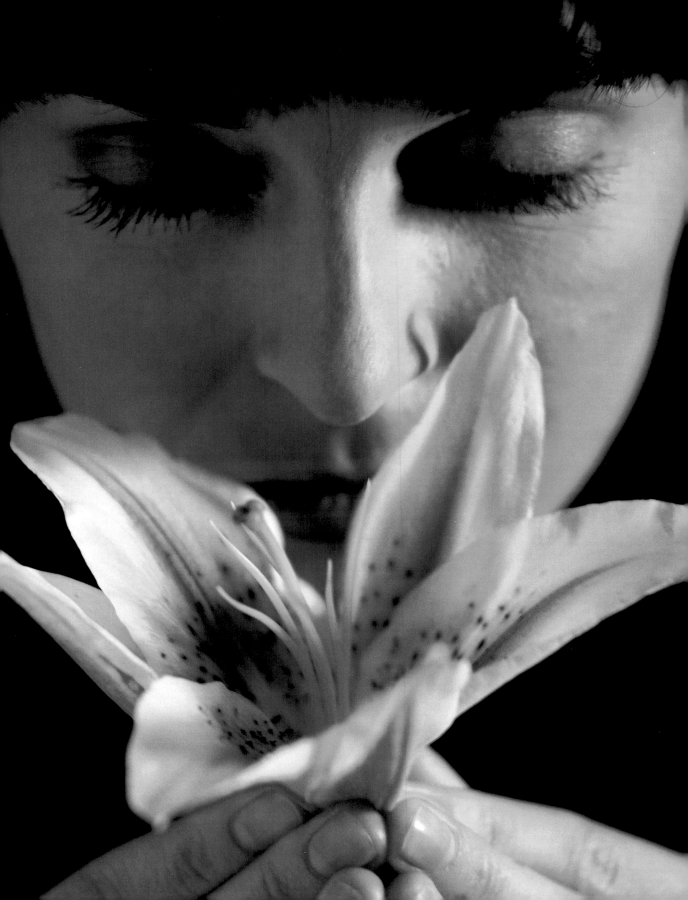

senses

'Kama is the enjoyment of appropriate objects by the five senses of hearing, feeling, seeing, tasting and smelling, assisted by the mind together with the soul. The ingredient in this is a peculiar contact between the organ of sense and its object, and the consciousness of pleasure which arises from that contact is called Kama.'

Kama Sutra

Through our five senses we experience the world and receive the pleasures it has to offer. All of us know the delight of biting into our favourite food or listening to a great song. The whiff of a familiar scent can conjure up a forgotten moment in time; the sight of a loved one or a beautiful landscape can move our emotions. The gentlest touch or an all-embracing hug can stimulate feelings of warmth and belonging, while the feel of your lover's bare skin against your own can be highly arousing. The *Kama Sutra* suggests many ways of stimulating the senses to heighten well-being and increase sexual appetite, from entertaining your lover with music to feeding them aphrodisiac foods or adorning them with flowers.

Touch

'He should touch her with his hands in various places,
and gently manipulate various parts of the body.'
Kama Sutra

The feelings we receive through touching and being touched are perhaps the most important of all the senses utilized within the *Kama Sutra*. Touch is the basis for how we explore and stimulate our own body and our lover's. The messages that our nerve endings transmit to our mind determine the strength and direction of our sensual pleasures. Emotions can be channelled through the hands to your lover, transferring an energy which is thought by many to have a healing quality.

In moments of intimacy, begin by gently touching using one finger or all your fingertips, the palm and the back of your hand, the nails to tickle the skin, and the knuckles to knead different parts of the back and legs. Slowly build up your own pattern for touching. Take it in turns to explore each other's body and tell one another what you like and want. Try using various objects to touch and tickle your lover's skin, such as a downy glove, peacock feather or ice cube. See how they respond to different textures.

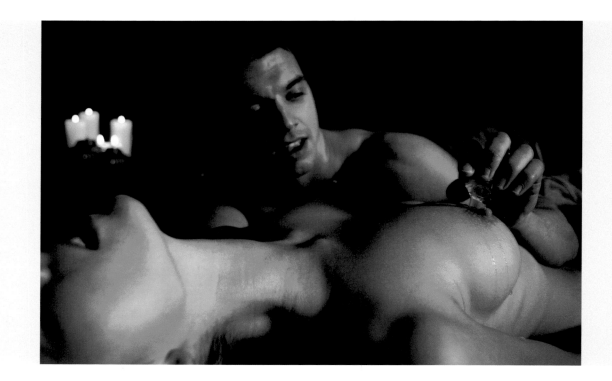

The man may like to have his loins stroked, to feel the woman's hair draped across his skin, her legs entwined with his, or her breasts pressed against him. The woman may enjoy being massaged with particular shiatsu or 'finger presses' to her head, shoulders, back and feet. She might prefer to lead her lover's hand over her body whilst he kisses her face, earlobes, neck, breasts, stomach and inner thigh. Or she may just like to be held in his arms.

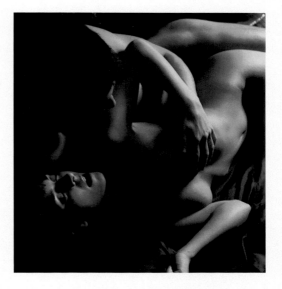

'...at the time of giving her some betel nut, or of receiving the same from her, or at the time of making an exchange of flowers, he should touch and press her private parts, thus bringing his efforts to a satisfactory conclusion.'

Kama Sutra

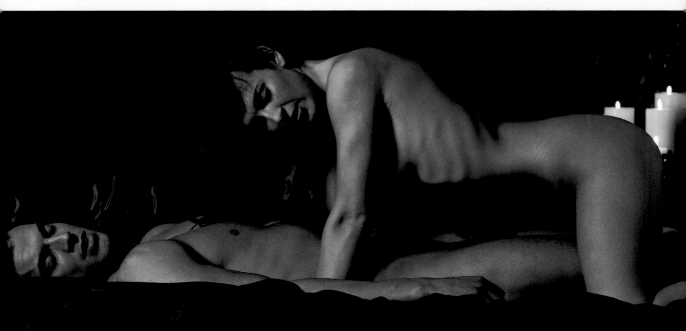

Taste

*'By eating the powder of the blue lotus, with ghee and honey,
a man becomes lovely in the eyes of others.'*

Kama Sutra

The *Kama Sutra* talks of many weird and wonderful recipes used to enhance lovemaking. Substances such as the oil of hogweed, the yellow amaranth, the leaf of the nymphae, peacock bones, and conch shells are all mentioned.

These archaic potions can be re-concocted with present-day ingredients known for increasing lust and passion, or for stimulating by their colour and shape. There are the phallic-shaped ginseng and mandrake roots, believed to hold restorative qualities; spices such as nutmeg, cinnamon and liquorice for increasing passion; fruits such as strawberries, grapes and cherries with their fleshy feel, sweet taste and sugar content for boosting energy. And of course, chocolate, forever the courting gift and rich in phenylethylamines, which trigger feelings of lust and satisfaction.

Food consumed or played with whilst naked will heighten your arousal. Try feeding one another; tantalize by keeping the morsel just beyond reach or spilling it purposefully. Ask your partner to close their eyes, or blindfold them, and get them to guess at foods by their taste, and vary the consistencies, hard or soft, sticky or runny.

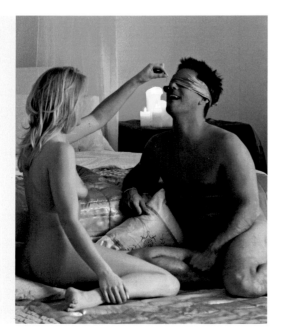

Food and Sex

Try placing different food – sweet dips, yoghurt, honey, cream – on sensitive parts of each other's body, then indulging yourselves slowly. Or work them into and over the skin, like massage oil, or even as a lubricant. The man pressing his mouth into a passion fruit or the woman slowly devouring a banana mimics the practice of oral sex and provides a visual thrill.

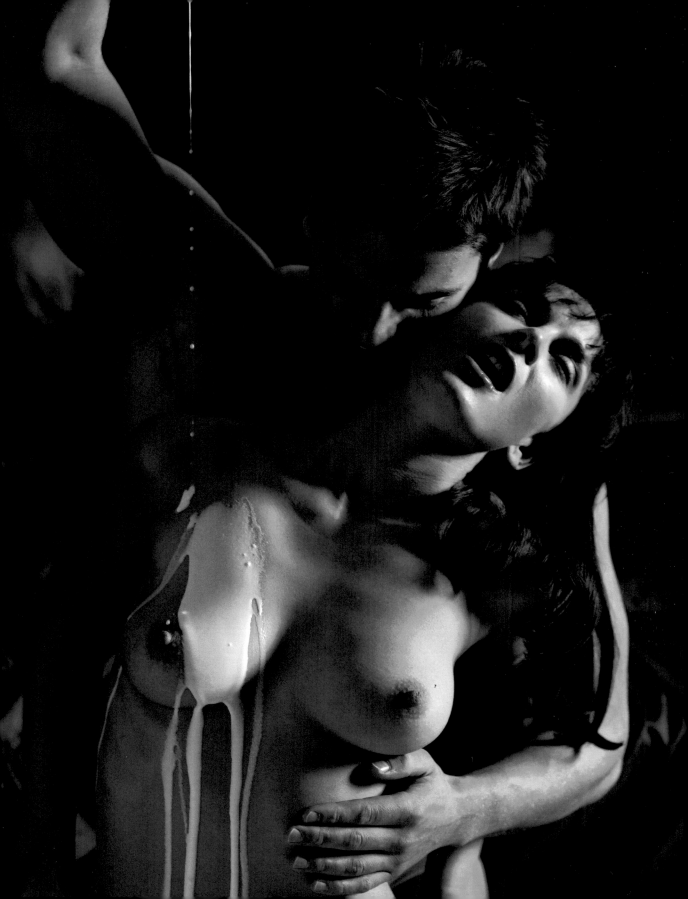

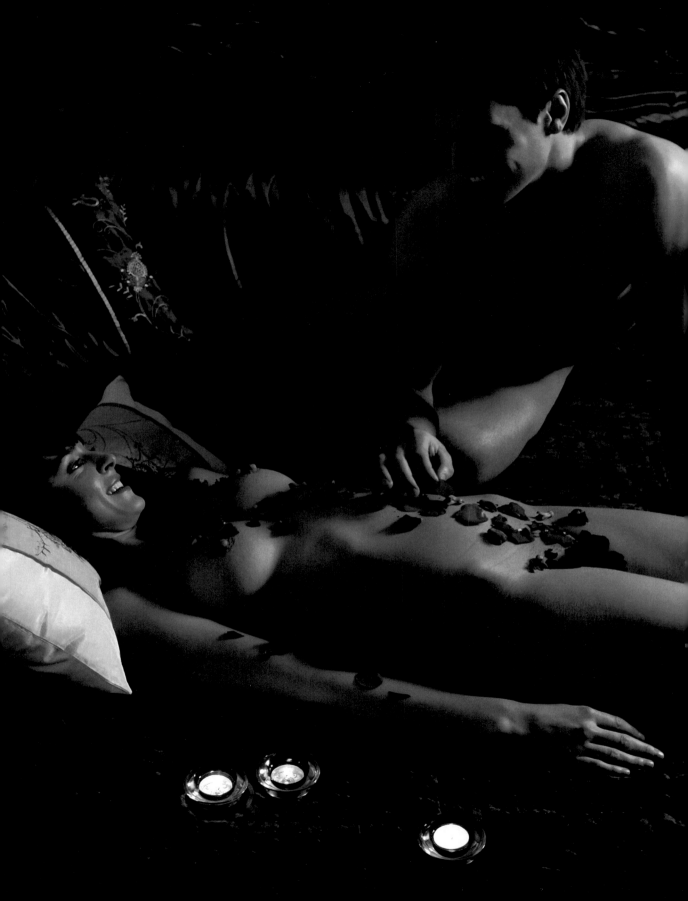

Smell

'The room, balmy with rich perfumes, should contain a bed, soft, agreeable to the sight, covered with a clean white cloth, low in the middle part, having garlands and bunches of flowers upon it. There should be also a couch besides, and at the head of this a stool, on which should be placed the fragrant ointments for the night, as well as flowers, pots containing collyrium and other fragrant substances, things used for perfuming the mouth, and the bark of the common citron tree.'

Kama Sutra

The smells surrounding us often enhance our mood and sometimes determine our sexual inclination. Just as a whiff of simmering food can bring on hunger, so the scent of certain perfumes and oils can arouse our passionate desire. The average human nose can detect about 4,000 different smells! Certain scents can bring back precise moments and sensations from our past. Because of this close link to our feelings, the ancient Indians deemed our sense of smell to be the most spiritual of all the senses.

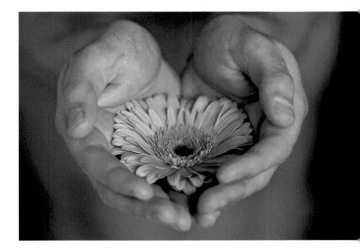

Surround yourselves with a pleasing fragrance, such as the aroma given off by scented candles or from burning essential oils, which will help to enhance the ambience. Choose a scent that is mutually pleasing. Jasmine and rose oil serve as strong aphrodisiacs, or there are the earthy fragrances of sandalwood and juniper which act as both stimulants and relaxants, whilst geranium oil or the exotic ylang ylang are known for their calming qualities. Scatter rose petals around the room and across your lover's body or fill the room with freshly cut flowers.

It has been shown that humans, after prolonged exposure to one another, release a chemical substance, or pheromone, that serves as a signature scent and may even work as a sexual enticement. It is important that you feel comfortable and relaxed with each other's unique scent and take pleasure in it. During lovemaking you will find that pheromones are released more strongly, providing a natural elixir.

Sight

'A man, who has seen and perceived the feelings of the girl towards him, and who has noticed the outward signs and movements by which those feelings are expressed, should do everything in his power to effect a union with her.'
Kama Sutra

Sight is perhaps our principal way of appreciating a potential partner, and many of the initial signs of attraction are visual ones. We look a little longer than usual, with our eyes a little wider open, and we check out different parts of the other person's body. The *Kama Sutra* talks of women turning away from their lover's eyes should they become overwhelmed. *'She never looks the man in the face, and becomes abashed when she is looked at by him; she looks secretly at him though he is gone away from her side.'*

Much of foreplay is about looking closely at one another and becoming aroused by what we see. During intercourse maintaining eye contact is essential, and feasting your eyes on your lover's body whilst you writhe together heightens your arousal and fills your mind with sensational images.

In varying degrees, men and women fuel their desires with sexual imagery. Men commonly use a visual stimulus when masturbating, and many women, whilst often visually stimulated too, find reading an erotic novel stimulates their imagination and can be a real turn-on. Some couples like to watch porn to get in the mood, or even whilst they do it on the sofa. If you have a camcorder, try videoing yourselves having sex (as long as you're both in agreement!) and use the sight of your own lovemaking as a means of arousal next time.

Being an unseen voyeur also feels elicit and exciting. Some couples get off on watching their neighbours having sex, whilst others like to be the exhibitionists, leaving their curtains open and their lights on to allow their lovemaking to be enjoyed by others.

Private Dancer

Perform a private striptease for your lover by slowly removing items of clothing, perhaps surreptitiously at first so that they are hardly aware of what you are doing, and then more obviously and erotically once they realize.
You can then become the audience as they return the favour by performing the same sexy routine for you.

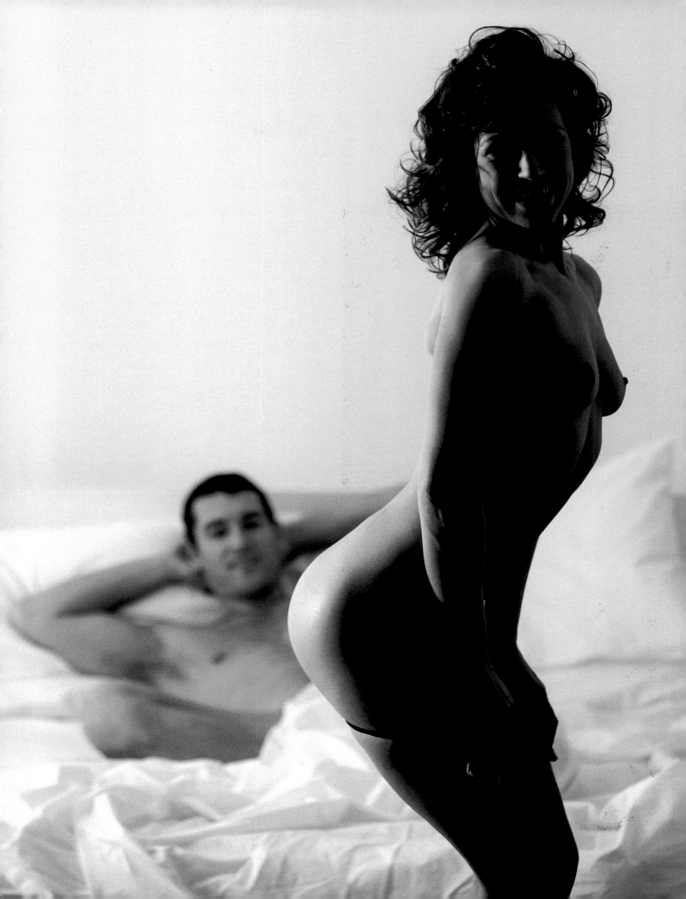

Sound

'Though a man loves a girl ever so much, he never succeeds
in winning her without a great deal of talking.'
Kama Sutra

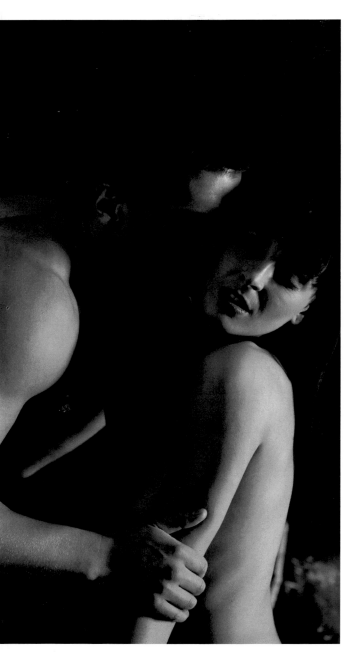

Our emotions are strongly stirred by everyday sounds, and we often use music to relax us or set the right atmosphere. The *Ananga Ranga* suggests scattering musical instruments, especially the pipe and the lute, about the place and singing amorous songs to one another. By comparison, many modern-day couples build up a repertoire of favourite songs to seduce and make love to. When heard again in public, these songs make them smile to each other at their secret significance.

Having sex outdoors can also be a great feeling. Listening to the sounds of birdsong, rushing water or the wind in the grass while you have sex can be intoxicating. Being at one with nature is a primal instinct, and you might find having a delicious picnic a good way of building up to a prolonged lovemaking session in the open air.

The physical sounds of sex – the squelching and slapping of our bodies – are powerfully erotic auditory sensations which increase our sexual responses. Most men like to hear, and get even more turned on by, the sound of their lover enjoying herself, whilst some women who moan out loud during sex are as turned on by their own noises. For some couples, talking dirty is another stimulus, either before or during sex.

Breathing as One

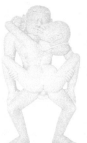

'When either of the lovers touches the mouth, the eyes and the forehead of the other with his or her own, it is called the Lalatika or "embrace of the forehead".' Kama Sutra

Breathing techniques can be used to increase intimacy between partners at any stage during lovemaking. Focusing on your breathing helps to 'centre' you and make you fully conscious of the moment and not distracted by unnecessary thoughts (such as what you need to do at work the next day, or what you would like for supper!). Taking deep breaths also helps to relax your entire body and produces a feeling of calm and well-being that seems to rise up from your very core. Holding your breath just before the moment of climax can make the experience even more intense.

Many different breathing and visualisation techniques are used in Tantric sex to help link your energy with your partner's:

- Sit close together facing each other and stare deep into each other's eyes. Feel as if you are looking into the very heart of your lover's being. Then close your eyes, breathe deeply and slowly, and focus on each inhalation and exhalation of breath.
- Let your breath begin to move in time with your lover's, imagining that it is like the rise and fall of a wave. As your breathing naturally falls into sync, you will feel at one with each other and enveloped by love and desire.
- When you feel ready, open your eyes and smile at your lover, acknowledging the warmth that you feel for each other, and embrace.

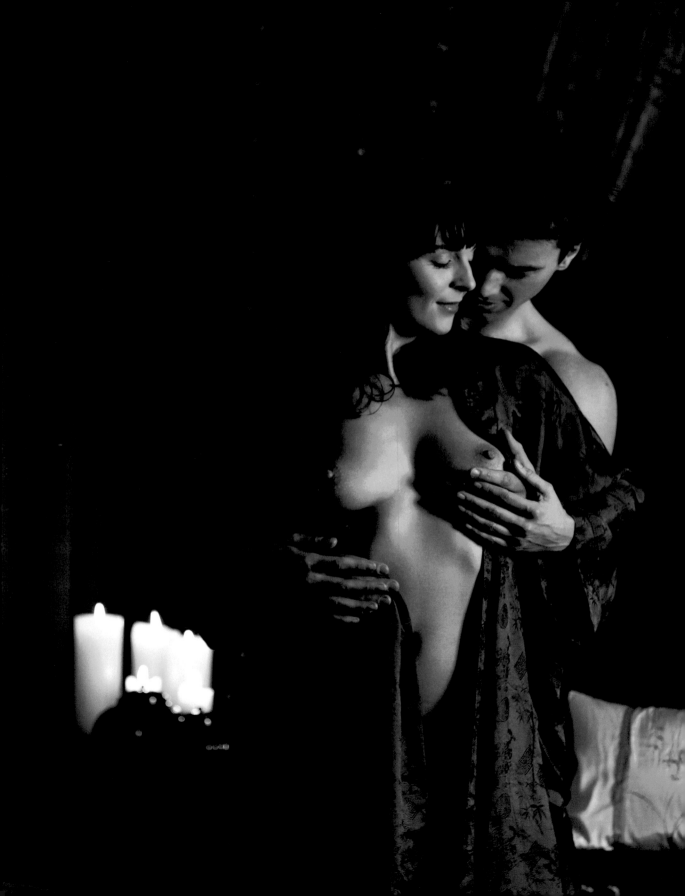

foreplay

'Women being of a tender nature want tender beginnings...the man should therefore approach the girl according to her liking, and should make use of those devices by which he may be able to establish himself more and more into her confidence.'

Kama Sutra

Many people think of lovemaking as intercourse but real sexual union, as taught by the *Kama Sutra* and other ancient texts, begins long before penetration. Foreplay is often an unfulfilled, sometimes overlooked part of the arts of loving, but the longer the rehearsal the better the final act. Foreplay is about translating our erotic thoughts and fantasies into actions; about heightening our desires yet teasing by restraint; and above all about slow-burning desire, as there is no better means of arousal than expectation.

Undressing

'He should loosen her girdle and the knot of her dress, and turning up her lower garment should massage the joints of her naked thighs, but he should not at that time begin actual congress.'

Kama Sutra

Shedding your clothes in the build-up to sex is often done swiftly as a routine act but it can be a wonderful introduction to foreplay if done slowly and seductively. Undressing one another with the eyes has long been an initial means of attraction; a figure-hugging outfit or an unbuttoned shirt draws our eye and encourages our curiosity. We imagine what lies beneath and fantasy quickly takes over.

The way we undress ourselves and each other displays obvious signs about our needs or intentions. Peeling your clothes off slowly can suggest a long session of languid sex is in store, whilst stripping quickly and forcefully shows a lustful passion.

Many people use clothing or outfits as part of foreplay. Provocative underwear is a firm favourite but it can also be fun and stimulating to wear different costumes or even cross-dress. Try on each other's underwear or stand naked apart from a tie or belt or high-heeled shoes. The woman might like to see her man with make-up on whilst he might find it kinky to see her in his favourite sports shirt.

The *Kama Sutra* talks of eunuchs disguised as bashful females with false breasts, and members of the royal harem dressing their maidservants like men. If role-playing or cross-dressing yourselves, instead of (or as well as) wearing costumes, try adopting different personas, or take it in turns to be the teacher and the pupil. This allows you to lose your inhibitions and say or demand things you may otherwise not feel comfortable with.

Try talking dirty, spanking or tying up your lover and blindfolding them. Fantasies build on the trust and intimacy between you, allowing your imagination and desires to run wild – often revealing hidden areas to your character in the process, which can be stimulating in itself.

Imagination and Anticipation

Calling your lover on the phone during the day, telling them in explicit detail what you are going to do to them later can be a real turn-on, letting your imagination run wild in anticipation of sex.

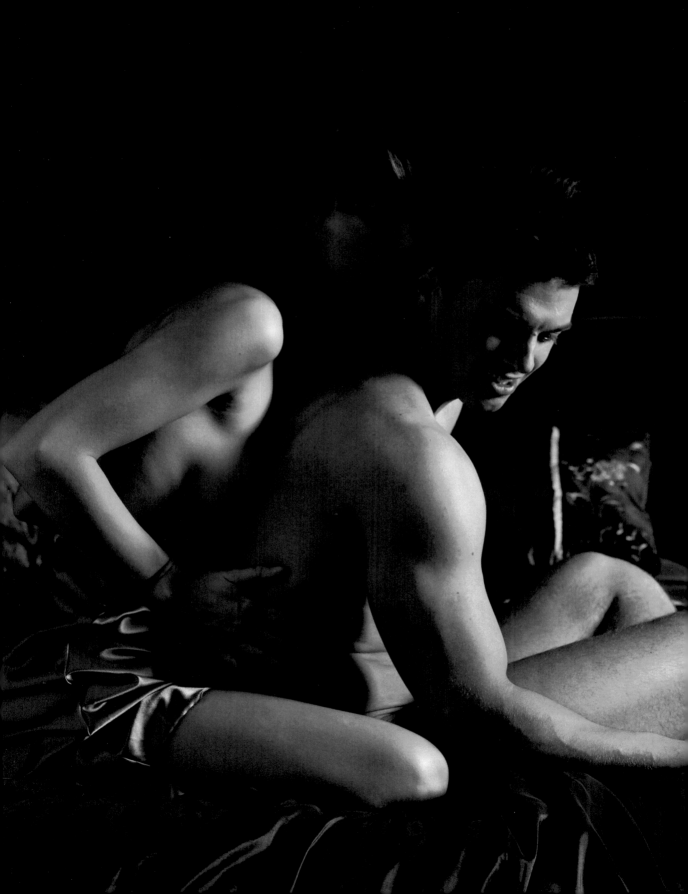

Kissing

'The wife, closing her husband's eyes with her hands, and closing her own eyes, thrusts her tongue into his mouth, moving it to and fro with a motion so pleasant and slow that it at once suggests another and higher form of enjoyment.'

Ananga Ranga

Kissing is an integral part of lovemaking and one of the most intimate ways in which we communicate our feelings for one another. It is our first form of sexual contact, often after a tantalizing build-up of suggestive gestures and prolonged eye contact.

The *Kama Sutra* says that a man should kiss his lover on the mouth softly and gracefully without making any sound, and that by achieving this he will have won her over and unlocked her passion and desire. There is no doubt that when you have experienced a wonderful kiss, it leaves you begging for more.

Body Kisses

Ask your lover to close their eyes then tease them with kisses on different parts of their body, everything from a peck to a bite. Begin slowly, kissing each part as if you were worshipping it, then build up the tempo until their body is throbbing with desire.

Oral hygiene is essential to the enjoyment of kissing; there is nothing more likely to make your lover recoil than bad breath. The *Kama Sutra* instructs men and women to keep their mouths 'tidy, sweet and clean' and it is a sign of consideration to your lover to approach them with fresh breath.

From a gentle brush of the lips to a deep, intense entwining of tongues, there are so many ways to kiss and, as with everything, variety is the key. Start off gently and be responsive to each other, taking it in turns to call the shots and dictate the rhythm. Pull back teasingly now and again to make your lover hot with desire then reconnect forcefully with their mouth, feeling their hot breath mingling with yours. A passionate kiss, where lovers are giving and receiving in equal measure and responding instinctively to each other's pressing and releasing, can create a powerful sense of fusion, so much so that you feel like you want to be swallowed up by your lover.

With their sensitivity and fleshiness, our lips, mouths and tongues resemble our sexual organs. When kissing, you can imagine that

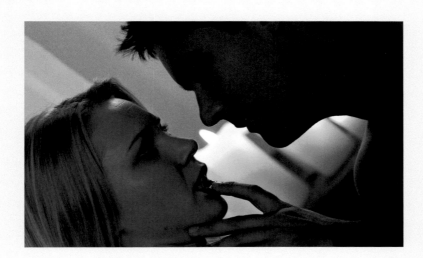

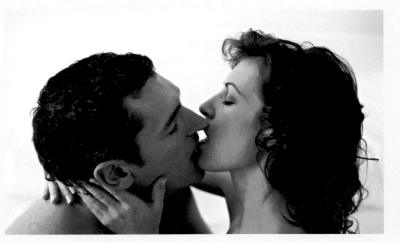

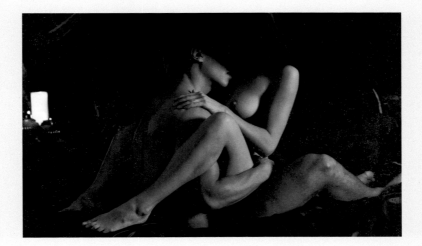

you are imitating intercourse: the tongue is the penis that pushes and probes; the lips the most sensitive part of the vulva. An especially potent kiss is known as *Uttarachumbita*, or the kiss of the upper lip. The man sucks gently on the woman's top lip, while she in turn kisses his lower lip. Using his tongue and lower lip, he gently rubs her frenulum, the small piece of connective tissue between the upper lip and the gum. This is believed to be a direct channel to the clitoris. Playing with it is likely to create a delicious tingling sensation in her genitals and, in some cases, can even lead to orgasm.

But it is not only our lips that are worthy of a kiss. The *Kama Sutra* recommends that we pay attention to the forehead, the eyes, the cheeks, the throat, the chest, and the breasts, and to vary the pressure depending on which of these you are kissing.

The *Kama Sutra* describes a game played with mouths where a wager can be laid as to who will get hold of the other's lips first. 'If the woman loses she should pretend to cry, should keep her lover off by shaking her hands and turn away from him.' In what is clearly another form of foreplay, it goes on to say that she should wait until her lover 'is off his guard or asleep, then get hold of his lower lip and hold it in her teeth, so that it should not slip away'. Furthermore she should celebrate her win by 'laughing and making a loud noise, deriding him, and dancing about, saying whatever she likes in a joking way, whilst moving her eyebrows and rolling her eyes'.

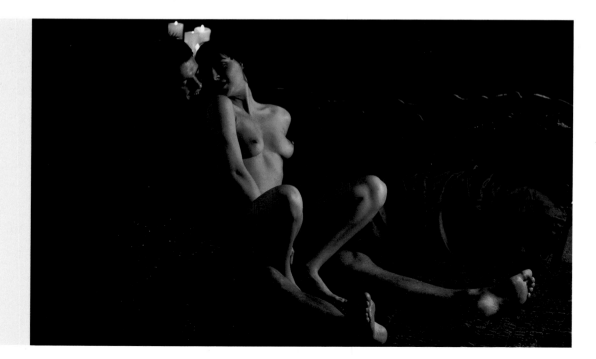

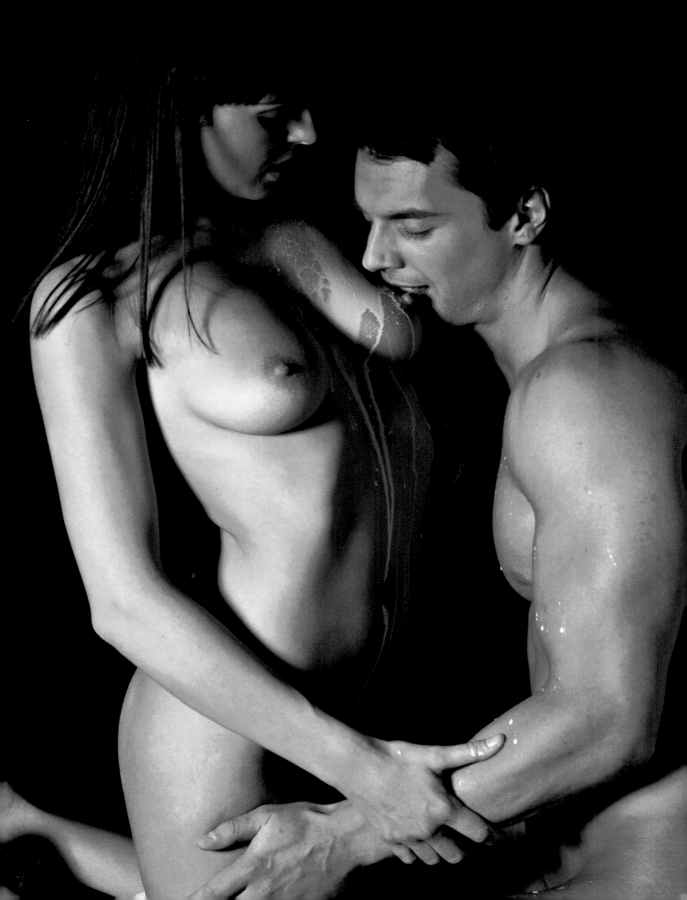

Embracing

'When two lovers are walking slowly together, either in the dark, or in a place of public resort, or in a lonely place, and rub their bodies against each other, it is called a "rubbing embrace".'

Kama Sutra

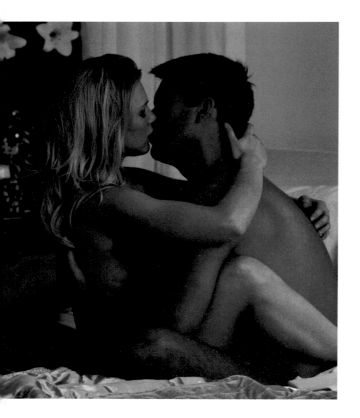

A full kiss is not complete without a loving embrace. Holding each other in our arms displays comfort and acceptance, as well as being a natural sign of affection. It appeals to our most primal instincts as we remember the warm and protective feeling of being cocooned in a parent's loving arms.

During foreplay we begin to entwine and press our bodies together, and, as ever, the slower the better. A good start is to stand facing one another with your toes and forehead touching and then to gradually press your thighs, belly and breasts together. This Tantric method allows energy to pass between the different points of contact and will be enhanced by closing your eyes, encircling each other with your arms and synchronizing your breathing.

The *Kama Sutra* describes many distinct embraces that indicate the mutual love of a man and woman. These vary in intensity from the initial flirtatious encounters of touching and 'piercing', where the lovers lightly brush against each other, to the titillation of rubbing and pressing, where their actions are more deliberate and passionate. As the heat rises, the woman clasps her lover like the 'twining of a creeper' or pulls herself towards him for a kiss, like the 'climbing of a tree'. Finally, when the lovers are so fired up that they are ready for intercourse, they should embrace as if they were entering into each other's body, becoming like a 'mixture of milk and water'.

Masturbation

Masturbation is one of the central elements of foreplay, and is often enjoyed as a separate pleasure altogether without leading to intercourse. It takes many forms and undoubtedly leads to better sex, by increasing your drive and desire. It is also a great relaxant, helping us to unwind and relieving us of stress and tension. Above all, it allows us to explore and experiment with our sexuality, teaching us how to maintain and prolong arousal.

Male Masturbation

'Before he engages in the final union with the woman, he should at the beginning excite his own passion by manually effecting erection. In this way he will activate his own passion and also be able to satisfy the woman.'

Kama Sutra

For centuries male masturbation was a taboo subject. Men wasting their semen, their life force, were seen to have committed a moral crime. Hindus believed that semen emanated from the blood and that the body needed a month or more to create one drop, so non-coital ejaculation was frowned upon.

Although the *Kama Sutra* makes little mention of masturbation, it does recommend it as a means of arousing passion.

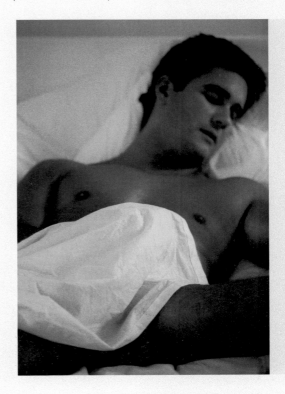

Masturbation is often fuelled by fantasy, and the thought of touching your body can be arousing in itself. Using both hands allows you to stimulate different areas simultaneously, such as caressing the testicles or rubbing the perineum whilst you masturbate. Try pinching the base of the shaft with one hand and with the other rub the glans with your fingertips placed downward, as if holding a tap. Some men like to simulate penetrative sex by pressing both palms against the shaft to mimic the walls of the vagina. Try this when standing in the shower: use a well-lathered sponge to squeeze the penis, then thrust into it.

Female Masturbation

The Hindus believed that the female genitals were the source of life-giving sexual energy and that the unlocking of this vital force was essential for sexual, physical and mental wellbeing. Various techniques for rubbing the yoni were recommended so it can be seen that women were not given such a hard time about masturbation as men!

When masturbating, fantasy is key to a woman's arousal, so relax and let your imagination go. Let the bathroom become your erotic chamber. Rub yourself along a towel draped over the edge of a bath or use the variable pressure of warm water from the showerhead to tease and tingle your vagina. Lying in a scented bath whilst you play with yourself is highly satisfying, as you feel enveloped by warmth and luxury. Deepening your breathing will help you relax and transport you to your very own realm of pleasure.

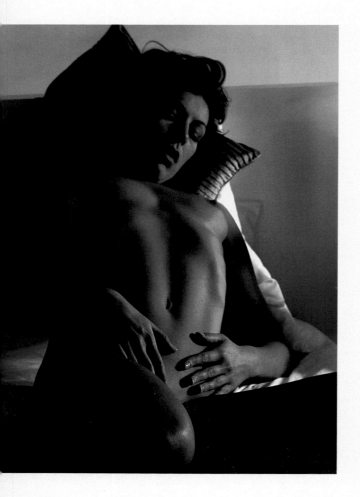

One technique is to form a V-shape with your index and forefinger and, whilst pressing down on your labia, close the fingers now and again to create a delightful squeeze on the clitoris as it swells and makes your vagina throb.

As an alternative to your own hands and fingers, you can experiment with sex toys, as the *Kama Sutra* states the 'women of the royal harem' would do, and 'accomplish their objective by means of bulbs, roots and fruits having the form of the lingam, or they lie down upon the statue of a male figure, in which the lingam is visible and erect.' These bulbs and roots are simply archaic versions of today's dildoes and vibrators, which come in more shapes and sizes than you can dream of! Fruits are still used by women too, from the obvious penile simulation of a banana or cucumber, to the fleshy parts of a mango or kiwi being rubbed against the vulva.

Mutual Masturbation

'At the commencement he should rub her yoni with his hand or fingers, and not begin to have intercourse with her until she becomes excited, or experiences pleasure.'
Kama Sutra

The beauty of masturbating yourself is that you can cast off all your inhibitions and indulge your deepest fantasies, explore the nuances of your body and find out just what turns you on. You may find that your orgasms are even more intense this way, as you control the pace and know all the right buttons to press. But masturbation should not be something that you do only when you are alone. Stimulating yourself in front of your lover is highly erotic and a good demonstration of exactly how you like to be touched.

Men Masturbating Women

Start by running your fingers along the woman's inner thighs teasingly, and gradually working your way towards her pubic mound. Once she is fully aroused, brush your fingertip ever so lightly across her labia, using a circular or side-to-side movement that skims the edge of the clitoris but does not stimulate it directly. Once she is wet, push your finger inside the entrance to the vagina and explore its unique fleshiness, while at the same time rubbing the clitoris gently with the base of your palm. Most men underestimate the sensitivity of the clitoris, so start gently and slowly, and above all, pay attention to her responses.

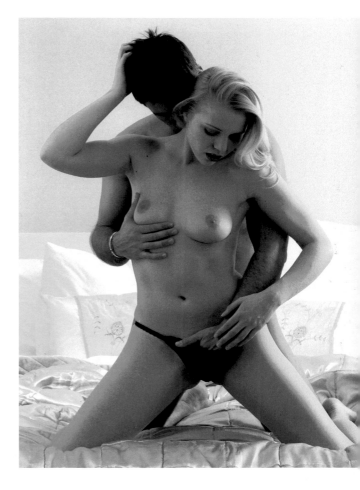

Masturbating each other can create a great closeness between you and is an exciting zone in which to experiment and explore. You need to spend time learning how to handle each other's genitals with tenderness and sensitivity. Tell each other what you like and guide your lover's hands.

Mutual masturbation is a great way to achieve simultaneous orgasm with your lover and helps to stir you up for a passionate session of sex. Lying on your backs whilst you pleasure each other is a restful pose which allows you to concentrate on the job in hand! The experience is further enhanced by the close eye contact you share and the intoxicating sound of your heavy breathing merging as you approach climax.

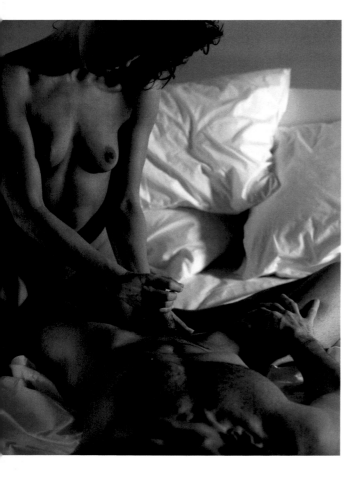

Women Masturbating Men

Start by holding the man's penis in the palm of your hand, gently squeezing it and rubbing the tip and ridge with your fingertips, luxuriating in the feel of his penis hardening in your hand as you toy with it.

Once erect, you can grip it with your entire hand or encircle it with a few fingers. From the most basic clenched fist, try using both hands every so often, or stopping at intervals to play with the tip and tease the small and highly sensitive urethral opening.

Sometimes the more friction the more intense the sensation, so form a ring with your thumb and forefinger and move it up and down loosely, letting your fingers catch the coronal rim of the head as you do so. Many women think that they need to be gentle all the time but once you have built up a steady rhythm, most men enjoy the pressure of your fingers remaining firm until they ejaculate.

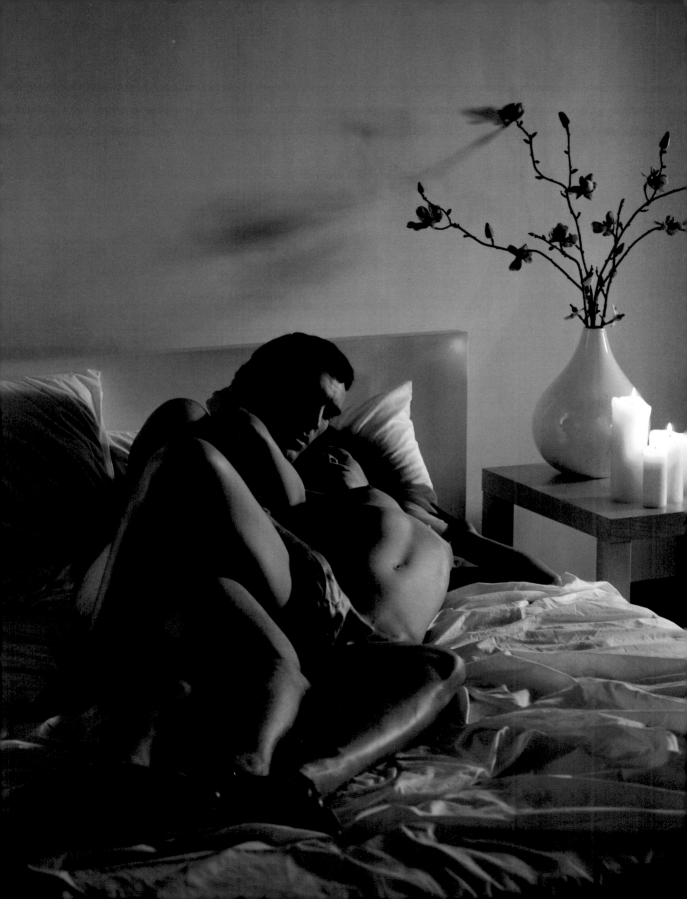

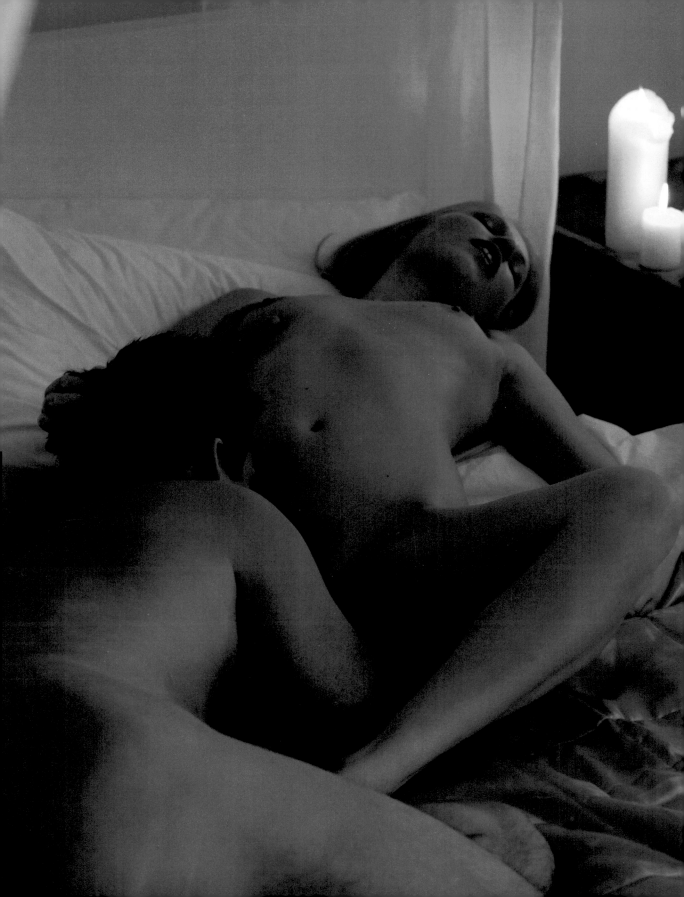

oral sex

'In some cases, oral congress is indulged in by a man and
and woman together, in which case, it should be done in the
same way as kissing.'

Kama Sutra

'Now spread, indeed cleave asunder, that archway
with your nose and let your tongue gently probe her
yoni with your nose, lips and chin slowly circling.'

Ratiratnapradipika

Oral sex is an intensely intimate experience, both physically and emotionally.
It can be used as part of foreplay prior to intercourse or as a complete act
in itself. Indeed, many people can have a very satisfying sex life based
around oral sex alone.

Relaxation and Intimacy

With its close mouth-to-genital contact, oral sex requires a good deal of trust and relaxation between partners. Without facial expressions to indicate enjoyment, it is important to tune in to the myriad but subtle physical cues that demonstrate the pleasure levels of your lover.

Cleanliness is vital to the enjoyment of oral sex so, if you have time, take a bath or shower with your lover beforehand. This has the added benefit of helping you to relax and unwind if you have had a busy day. While bad body odour can be a real turn-off, the natural juices that we emit from our genitals during sex can act as a powerful elixir and should be relished. As you get to know your lover more intimately, their individual aroma will become more and more familiar and intoxicating.

Alternatively, if carnal odours aren't your thing, all is not lost! You could try smearing yoghurt or chocolate spread or a fruit smoothie or any other food that you fancy over your lover's genitals to disguise their scent. You may wish to do this anyway, as it will add an element of fun and experimentation to your lovemaking. Remember that the more you laugh together, the more relaxed and open you will be.

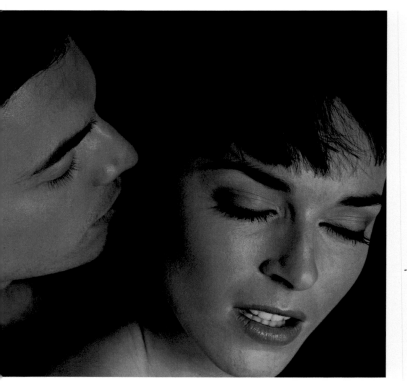

'With delicate fingertips, pinch the arched lips of her house of love very very slowly together, and kiss them as though kissing her lower lip.

'Let your tongue rest for a moment in the archway to the flower-bowed Lord's temple before entering into worship vigorously, causing her seed to flow....'

Ratiratnapradipika

Cunnilingus

'Some women of the harem, when they are amorous, do the acts of the mouth on the yonis of one another, and some men do the same thing with women. The way of doing this should be known from kissing the mouth.'

Kama Sutra

The *Kama Sutra* makes scant reference to cunnilingus, as it was not considered a proper act to be done by respected members of society, but Indian sculptures and poems suggest that it was certainly in vogue at some stage, and a later treatise on sex, the *Ratiratnapradipika* by Devaraja, mentions eight types of oral sex to be performed by men on women.

The clitoris is one of the most sensitive points on a woman's body and, if stimulated properly, she will feel sexually satisfied. Giving a woman such intense pleasure is equally fulfilling for the man so he should take time to find out exactly what she likes. The most comfortable position for the woman is to lie back on a bed, with the man lying between her legs. Placing a pillow beneath her buttocks will raise

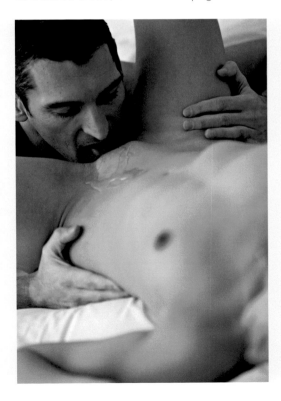 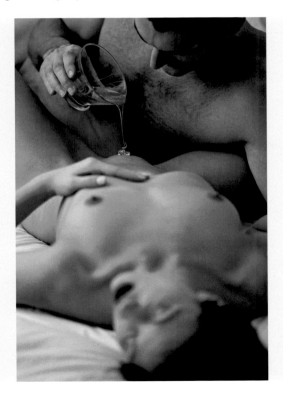

her pelvis, creating an easier angle for him. He could also kneel on the floor with the woman at the edge of a bed or sofa or even sit at the kitchen table and feast on her as if enjoying a banquet!

Women vary considerably in their likes and dislikes so it is important to read the messages that your lover gives to you. Obvious signs that a woman is enjoying what her partner is doing are: her pelvis and thighs relax, her breathing becomes heavier and she offers herself to your mouth more. If she is not comfortable, she will pull back or try to push your head away slightly. The clitoris itself also offers clues: if it enlarges, she likes what you are doing; if it shrinks she doesn't.

As most women like a build-up to sex, start by kissing her mouth, demonstrating what you might do on her genitals later. Slowly and seductively, you can work your way downward, kissing her neck, her nipples and her navel, then her inner thighs, sensing the slow build-up of excitement in your lover. Teasing her by lightly brushing her labia with your tongue is likely to bring her to an almost unbearable level of desire. Once she has reached this point, you can start to tantalize her clitoris with careful movements of the tongue, lips, teeth and fingers. You should never focus on the clitoris for too long, as over-stimulation is likely to make it lose sensitivity altogether and cause her discomfort (or even pain). By experimenting with different techniques on different parts of her genitals, and tuning in to her responses is guaranteed to prolong her arousal.

Using the tongue, make slow or fast circling movements on the tip or around the edge of the clitoris. Vary the direction to find out which she prefers. Up and down or side-to-side flicks are also highly pleasurable. Start with light brushes, only using harder flicks when the woman is fully aroused. Very carefully, take the clitoris between your teeth (if this is too much for the woman or her clitoris is not exposed enough, the lips can be used instead) to envelop it and bring it in closer contact with your tongue. Sucking it gently while circling or flicking your tongue across it will result in maximum arousal for the woman.

Lick her labia and the lower part of her vulva and alternate this with gentle pushes of your tongue inside the vagina. At the same time, you can rub your nose against her clitoris so that every part of her is stimulated. Use your fingers to part her labia gently and expose the clitoris or to explore the inside of her vagina. Try a back-and-forth motion just inside the vagina behind the clitoral area and alternate this with strokes of the clitoris with your tongue. Repeat this action several times, building up a rhythm of ecstasy for your lover. Anal stimulation during oral sex can also be highly arousing for some women, especially when they are close to climax.

If you sense that your lover is about to come, do not let go of her clitoris or try something different. Keep the pressure constant until she indicates that you can let go. There's nothing worse than being mid-orgasm and suddenly losing the stimulation.

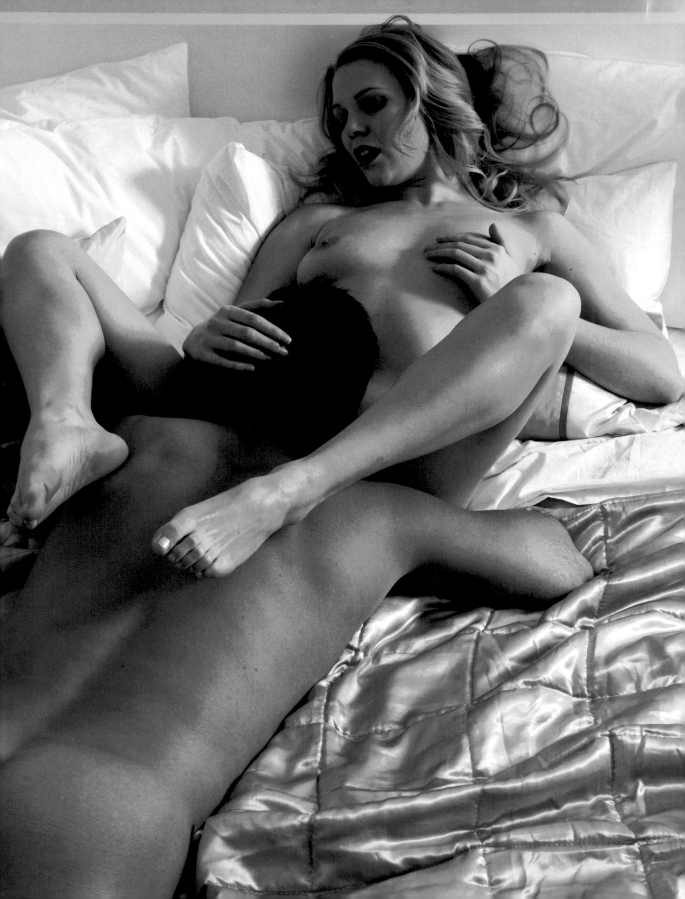

Fellatio

'When holding the man's lingam with her hand… and she puts the half of it into her mouth, and forcibly kisses and sucks it, this is called "sucking a mango".'
Kama Sutra

Nearly all men enjoy the feeling of a woman's mouth around their penis. The beauty of giving a man oral sex is that it can be performed in a number of places where full sex is a bit tricky, such as the office toilet, under a blanket in the park, or even on a long-distance flight! As with women, men vary in their preferences. The trick is to use a variety of techniques – slow, fast, deep, shallow, licking, sucking – to discover what he likes best.

In the spirit of *Kama Sutra*, start by concealing your desires, slowly massaging the man's thighs and working your way upward, gradually getting closer to his penis. The thought of what you are about to do is likely to fire him up, but tease him by stopping after each movement. Waiting until he is almost begging for more is likely to heighten the experience for him.

Hold his penis in your hand and gently caress it, whilst using your other hand to fondle his testicles, stroke his thighs or push against his perineum (the highly erogenous area between the anus and the scrotum). Look at him, licking your lips seductively, then run the head of his penis along your wet mouth and slap it gently against your tongue. Blow lightly on the tip and circle your tongue around the coronal ridge that separates the glans from the shaft. As he hardens, relax your grip so that you can run your flat tongue right up the length of his shaft. The sensitive area is on the underside of his penis, just below the head, so linger here for a while.

Take his penis into your mouth. Show him your enjoyment by murmuring as if you are sucking on your favourite sweet, or on a mango fruit, as the *Kama Sutra* suggests. This humming creates a vibration on the head of the penis, which some men enjoy. Vary how deep you take him into your mouth. If you don't like deep-throating, use your hands to encircle his shaft whilst you suck and lick the top. When you sense that he is near to climax, keep up a steady rhythm and do not vary the pressure, as this can be highly frustrating. Whether you decide to swallow or not is entirely your own preference. If you prefer to swallow, then keep a glass of ice-cubes in water handy, both for drinking afterwards, or for using the ice-cubes in your mouth or on his body. In a loving relationship you should always respect each other's wishes. Most men prefer to come in your mouth but letting him ejaculate over your breasts or stomach can be just as satisfying for him.

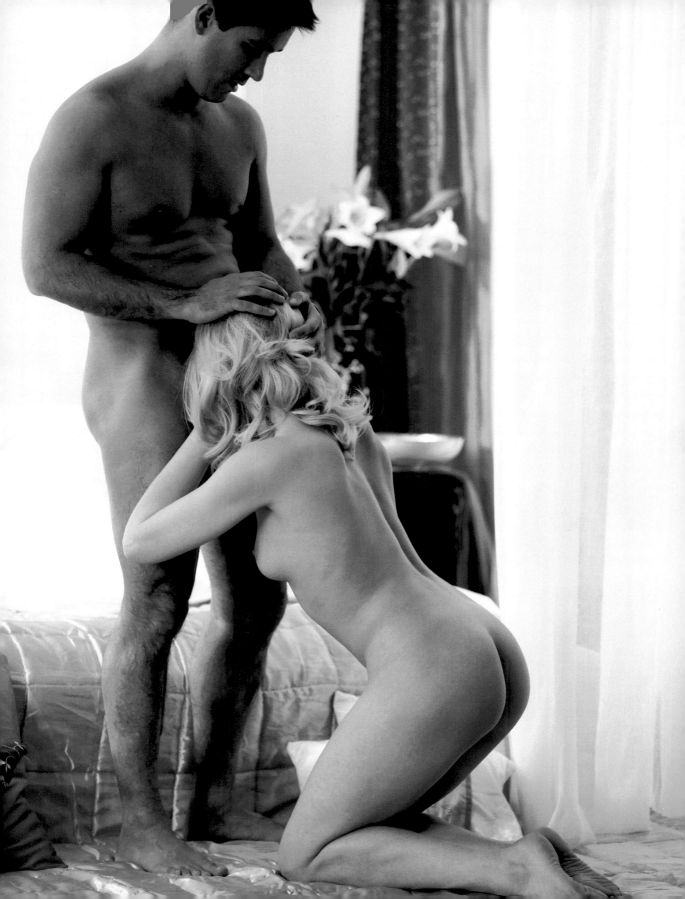

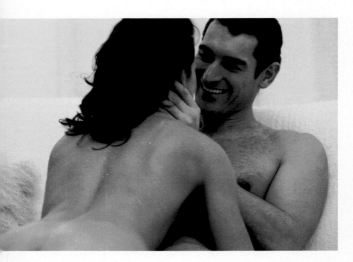

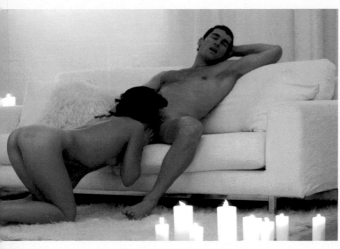

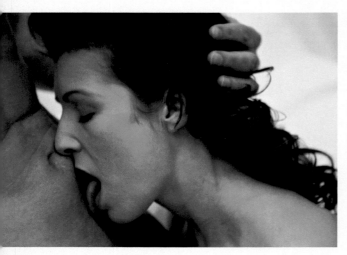

'Mouth Congress'

The *Kama Sutra* recommends eight ways of giving 'mouth congress', which should be performed in sequence:

1. **Nimita:** hold the man's penis with your hand, place it between your lips and move it about in your mouth.

2. **Parshvatodashta:** cover the end of the penis with your fingers collected together like the bud of a plant or flower, then press the sides of it with your lips and teeth.

3. **Bahih-Sandamsha:** press the head of the penis with your lips closed together and kiss it as if you were drawing it out.

4. **Antah-Sandamsha:** put the penis further into your mouth and press it with your lips and take it out again.

5. **Chumbitaka:** hold the penis in your hand and kiss it as if you were kissing your lover's lower lip.

6. **Parimrishtaka:** touch it with your tongue everywhere, and pass your tongue over the head.

7. **Amrachushitaka:** put it halfway into your mouth and kiss and suck it forcibly.

8. **Samgara:** put the whole penis into your mouth and press it to the very end as if you were going to swallow it up.

Sixty-nine

'When a man and a woman lie down in an inverted order, i.e. with the head of the one towards the feet of the other, and carry on this congress, it is called Kakila, "the congress of a crow".'

Kama Sutra

This famous way of having oral sex is the ultimate shared experience, in which you can enjoy the dual pleasure of giving and receiving. In *Kama Sutra* terms, it allows the Shiva and Shakti energies to flow freely between lovers at the same time, and the warmth that this generates can be highly gratifying.

The most common position is for the woman to straddle the man with her vagina close to his face. In this pose, his hands are free to hold her buttocks and stroke her sides or he can use his fingers to part her labia and expose her clitoris. As the angle is reversed, the woman can now use her upper lip and fingers to stimulate the sensitive underside of his penis. Alternatively, many couples find it easier and more relaxing to lie side-by-side, with the man's head resting between the woman's thighs. Try to match each other's rhythm or take it in turns to apply stimulation. Over time, you will be able to anticipate each other's responses and learn to bring each other to climax simultaneously.

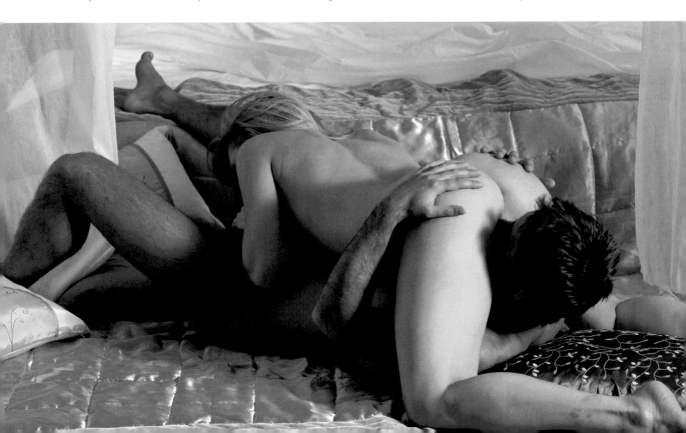

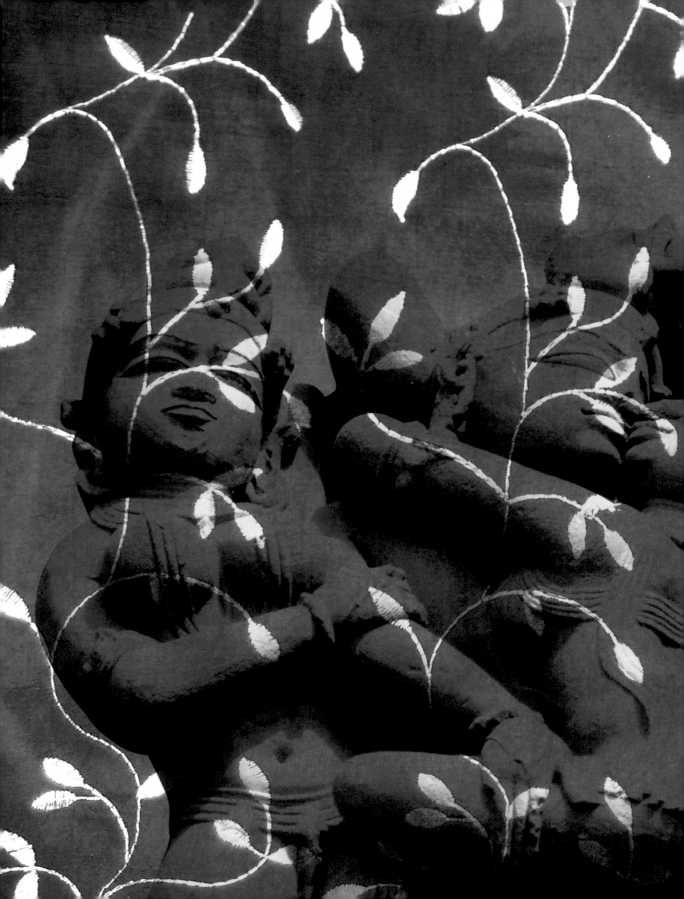

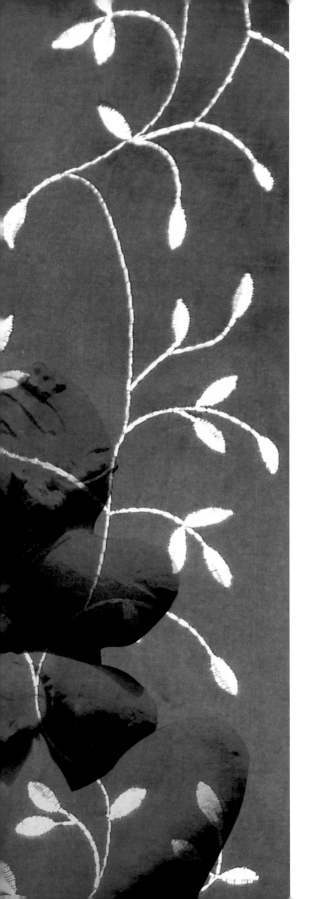

THE
KAMA
SUTRA

The Twining

'While the woman is lying on his bed, he should loosen the knot of her undergarments and overwhelm her with kisses. Then when his lingam is erect he should touch her with his hands in various places and gently manipulate various parts of the body. If the woman is bashful, and it is the first time that they have come together, the man should place his hands between her thighs.'

Kama Sutra

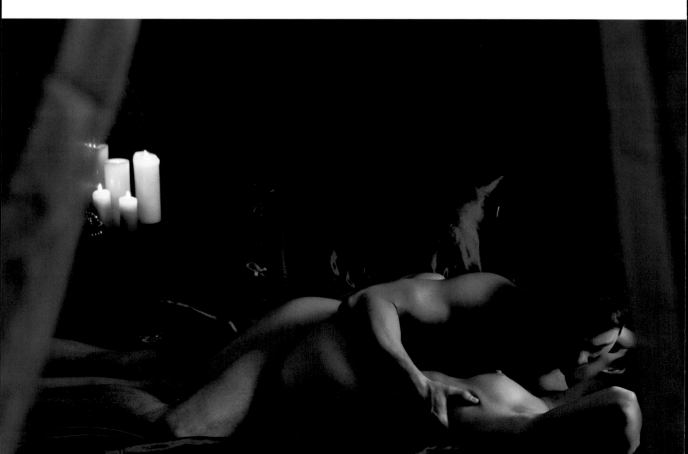

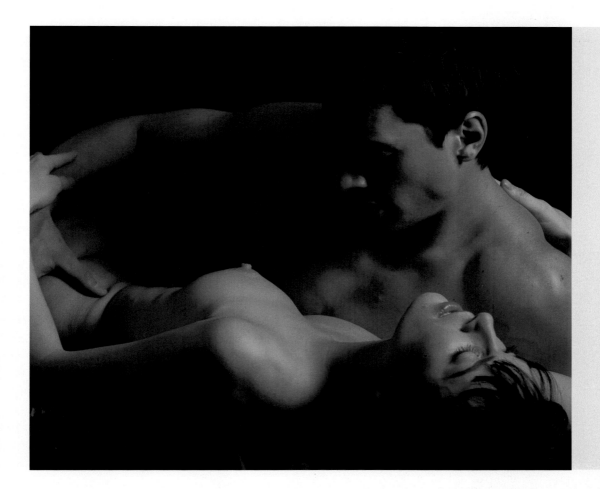

This is one of the first positions mentioned in the *Kama Sutra* and is an ideal one to start in, as it quickly builds up intimacy and arousal, and allows full body contact in a restful pose for both partners. Lie on your sides, facing one another. Looking deep into each other's eyes, your hands are free to caress and explore one another. Kiss each other gently and savour the sensuousness of your entangled bodies. Placing her upper thigh across her lover, the woman entwines him in a closer embrace and indicates that she is ready for him.

The man slips his penis slowly inside her vagina and, with gentle thrusts, he builds up a steady rhythm. The woman can alter the tightness of the clasp by raising or lowering her leg. Once the lovers are both well aroused and ready, the man, still between the woman's thighs, can raise himself up onto his knees while the woman remains supine.

DIFFICULTY	🌷 🌷 🌷 🌷
TYPE	soft, gentle, slow

The Yawning

'The signs of the enjoyment and satisfaction of the woman are as follows:
her body relaxes, she closes her eyes, she puts aside all bashfulness, and shows
increased willingness to unite the two organs as closely together as possible.'

Kama Sutra

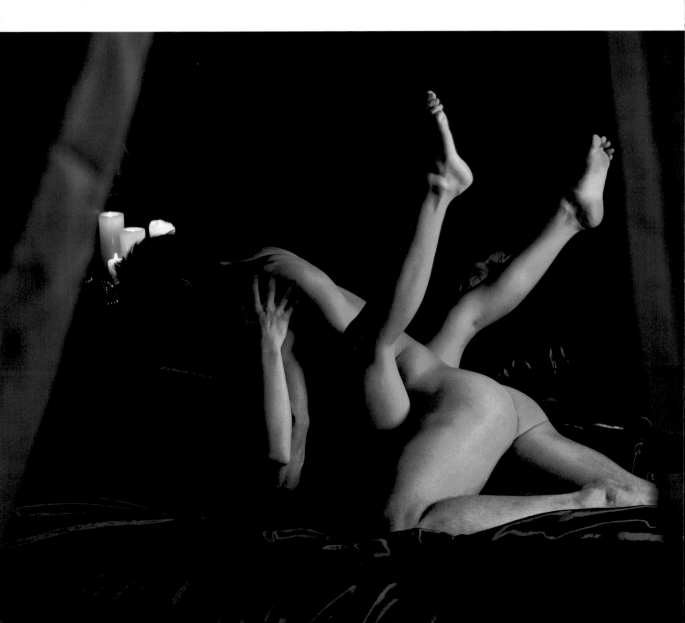

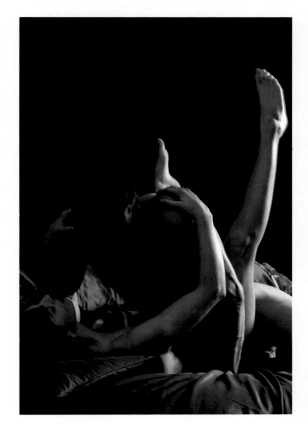

With the woman's legs raised and wide apart, or 'yawning', this is an effective and satisfying position for deep and intense penetration. The man leans over his lover in a dominant pose, resting on his hands, and supporting her thighs with his. Although he controls the thrusting, she may vary the sensation by changing the position of one or both her legs (she will probably want to do this anyway to avoid muscle ache!) or by pushing her pelvis forward. She might like to reach down and push her clitoris against his pulsing penis. The man can punctuate his thrusting by stopping to lean forward and kiss his lover deeply while she clenches him tightly with her legs.

DIFFICULTY	✿ ✿ ✿ ✿
TYPE	deep, intense

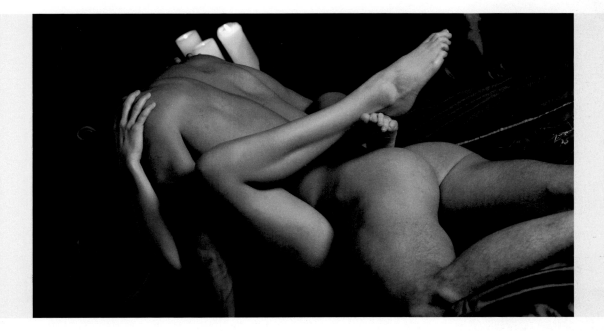

Splitting the Bamboo

VENUDARITAKA

The woman rests her ankles on the man's shoulders as he kneels with his thighs either side of her buttocks. He must enter her slowly as the vagina is shortened in this position. She places one foot on his chest (she can feel his heart beating through her toes) and alternates the position of her legs, allowing her to dance to her own rhythm.

She controls the pace whilst her lover remains still, observing her unfolding pleasure and resisting the urge to take control. The angle of this position or 'low congress' narrows the vagina so that, as she moves her legs, it rolls and squeezes him, providing a slow penis massage. Running his nails gently up and down her thighs as she 'dances' will give her a spine-tingling sensation.

DIFFICULTY				
TYPE		intense, slow		

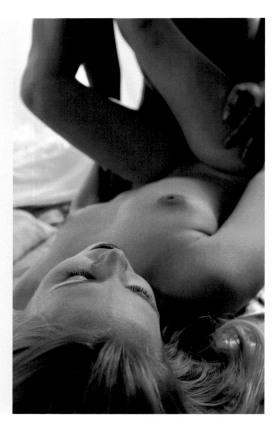

Kama Sutra Position Names

Often, the positions in the Kama Sutra have poetic, evocative names, such as Splitting the Bamboo, Sporting of a Swan or The Twining of a Creeper. All these positions are meant as pointers only and Vatsyayana recommends that you vary them according to your own liking.

As you experiment in your lovemaking and discover new positions that you both enjoy, why not create your own names for them? Be as fantastical or as romantic or as ridiculous as you like!

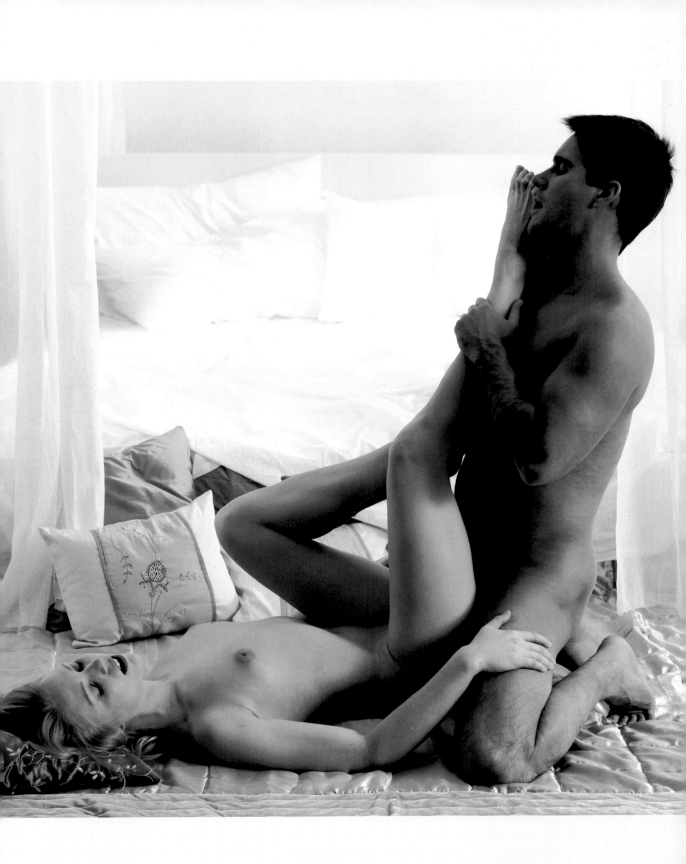

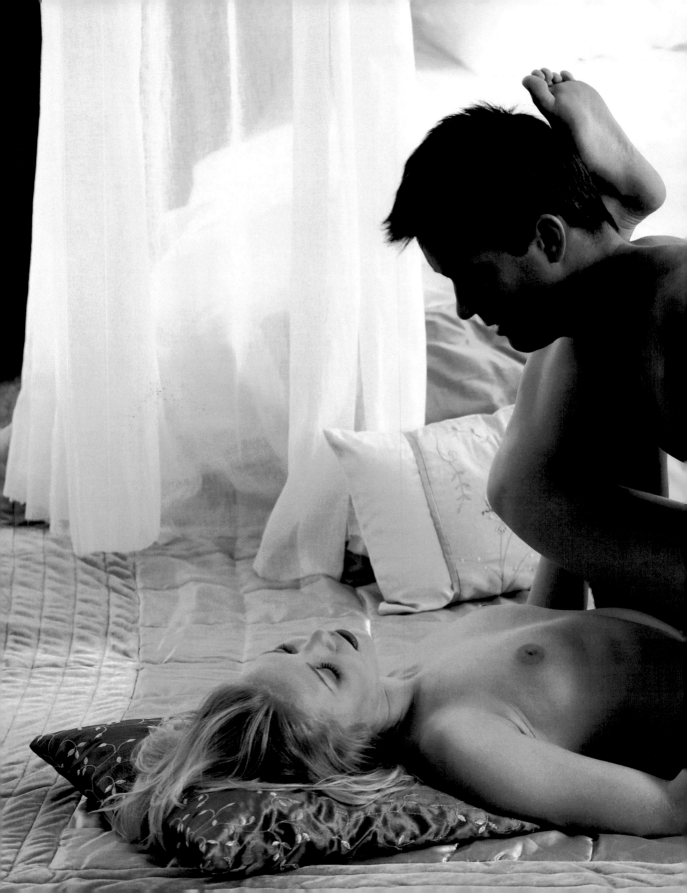

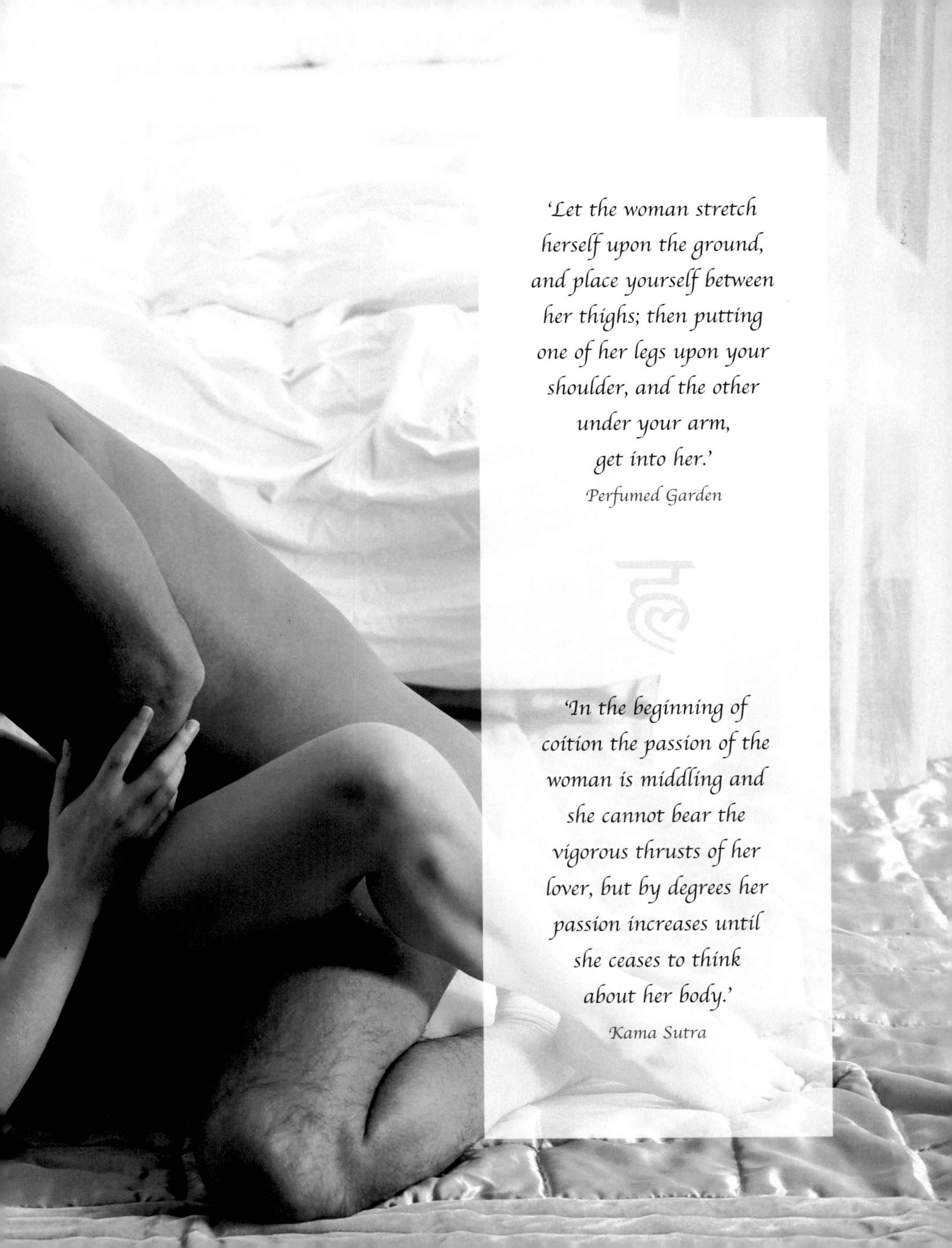

'Let the woman stretch
herself upon the ground,
and place yourself between
her thighs; then putting
one of her legs upon your
shoulder, and the other
under your arm,
get into her.'
Perfumed Garden

'In the beginning of
coition the passion of the
woman is middling and
she cannot bear the
vigorous thrusts of her
lover, but by degrees her
passion increases until
she ceases to think
about her body.'
Kama Sutra

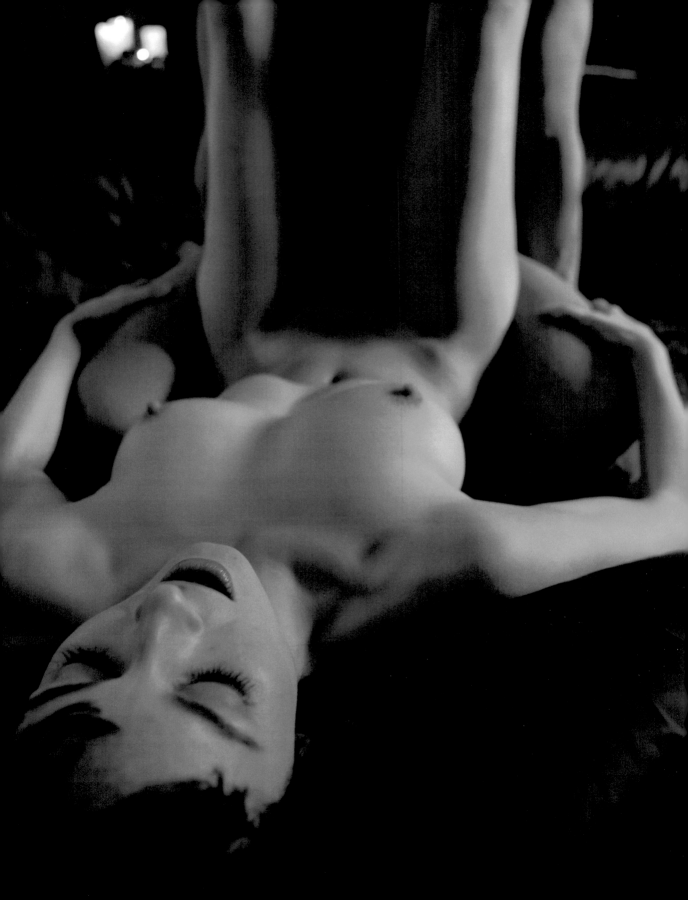

Genital Size

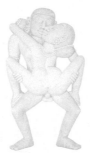

The *Kama Sutra* separates men into three types according to the size of their penis: the hare (small), the bull (medium) and the horse (large). Similarly, there are three types of woman – the deer, the mare and the elephant – depending on the depth of their vagina. This means that there are nine different types of union according to dimensions but only three where the lovers fit each other perfectly.

Obviously, the least satisfying scenario is a hare man with an elephant woman but a horse man with a deer woman is also not ideal. A woman may not know how deep her vagina extends but, if you have experienced the discomfort of a large penis pushing against your cervix, this will give some indication that you are not the largest size. You will find that some positions are more comfortable than others. Do whatever feels natural and don't worry if a particular position doesn't work for you.

When a man is larger than the woman, the *Kama Sutra* recommends positions that widen or lengthen the vagina, such as Vijrimbhitaka (The Yawning). When the man is smaller, positions such as Veshtitaka (The Twining) and Bhramaraka (The Spinning of the Top) are recommended, as the vagina is contracted, putting an extra squeeze on the penis.

The main message is to try out all the different positions and find out what is most enjoyable for you as a couple.

Pressing Passion

UTPIDITAKA

'The legs are contracted, and thus held by the lover before his bosom...'
Kama Sutra

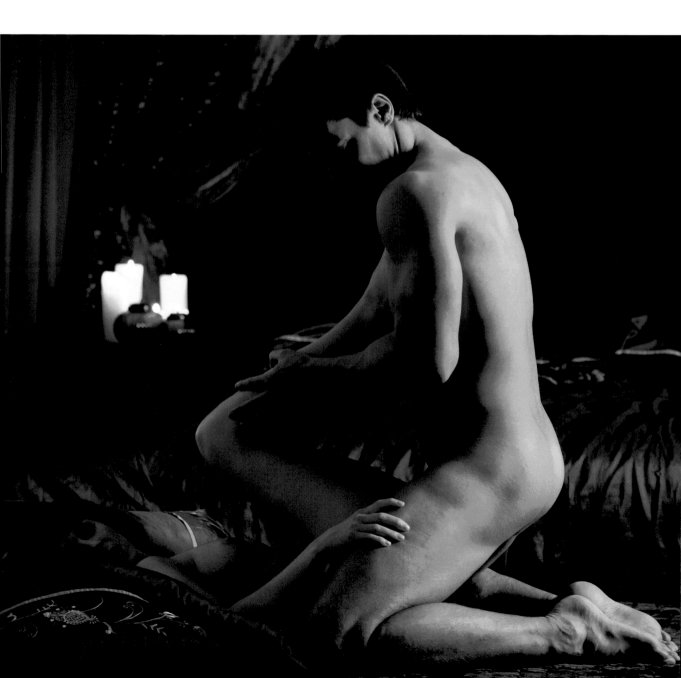

The woman raises both legs and places the soles of her feet on the man's chest, keeping her thighs together. She may enjoy having the man under her feet in this way! The man should take care when penetrating her, as the vagina is shortened and the sensation is intense.

The woman needs to be bold and tell her partner just what she likes and how far he can thrust without causing pain. If he is thrusting too hard, using her feet to apply pressure on his chest should give him the message! This is a good position for the man to partially withdraw intermittently to alter the depth and strength of his strokes before he penetrates her deeply once again.

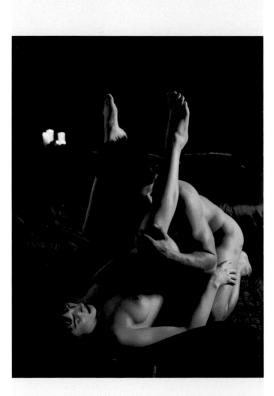

To vary the rhythm, the woman can move her hips from side to side while the man holds her knees together to help increase her grip on him. In a break from thrusting the man can concentrate for a moment on massaging his lover's calves, ankles and feet. Holding a foot in each hand, press the thumb firmly into the arches of her soles, working them in a clockwise and then anticlockwise fashion, and then slowly squeeze each toe with your thumb and forefinger.

DIFFICULTY	🌼 🌼 🌸 🌸
TYPE	deep, fast

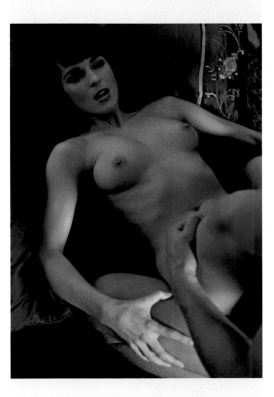

The Rising

The *Kama Sutra* recommends this position for the Hastini (or elephant-type of woman) only, as the vagina is much shortened in this pose and a smaller woman would be uncomfortable. The woman, enfolded within the man's thighs, raises her legs up high, keeping them tightly squeezed together. She holds onto his hips while he clasps her ankles or thighs. The man gently moves his penis in her vagina, using slow circular motions or soft thrusts while she lies still, enjoying the feel of him exploring her depths. This position could also be used immediately after orgasm as the woman can hold the penis as tightly as possible with her vagina, while the man kisses her feet and ankles in a gesture of adoration and devotion.

DIFFICULTY	☙ ☙ ☙ ☙
TYPE	soft, intense, slow

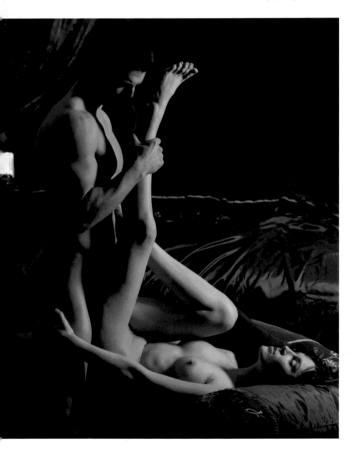

The Thrust

As it is the man who controls movement in this position, and because of his choice of angles, it is a good position for him to experiment in. Other eastern texts suggest different 'systems' of thrusting, both to maximise the woman's pleasure, and also to prolong penetration by carefully practised semen retention.

To help achieve this try a few shallow thrusts, where only the head of the penis enters the vagina, followed by a deeper one, and then the same in reverse. According to preference you will soon build up your own scale.

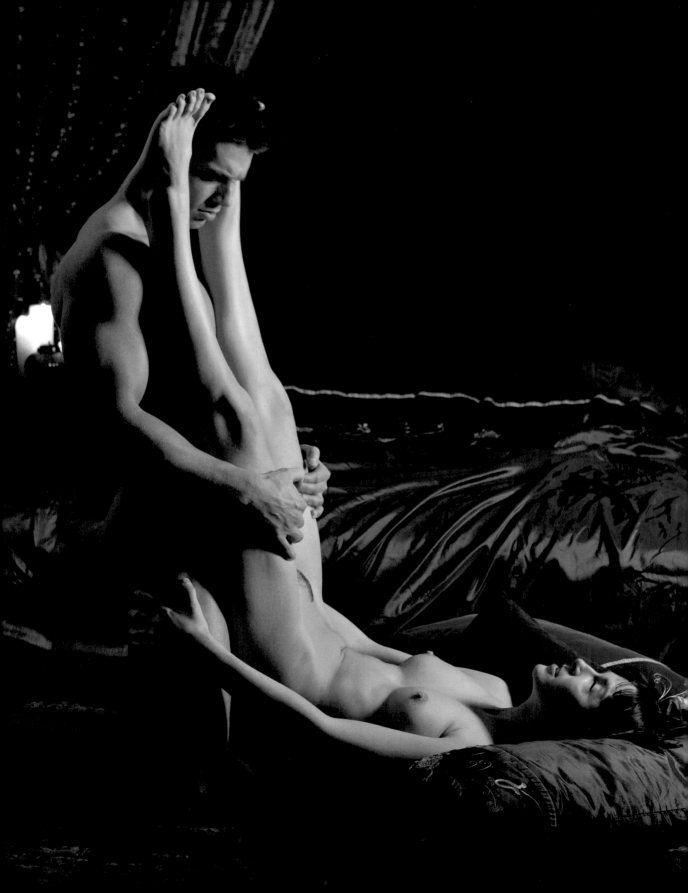

The Twining of a Creeper

JATAVESHTIKA

'When a woman, clinging to a man as a creeper twines round a tree,
bends his head down to hers with the desire of kissing him, and slightly makes
the sound of sut sut, embraces him, and looks lovingly towards him, it is called
an embrace like the jataveshtika or twining of a creeper.'

Kama Sutra

This position can be moved into quickly if your desire is urgent, but is also good for gentleness. The woman sits opposite her lover on the edge of the bed. The man squats down and, pushing her legs apart, runs his fingers up and down her thighs.

This is a highly erogenous zone so he will enjoy watching her excitement rise again until it reaches almost boiling point. The woman squats over him and, taking his penis in her hand, she guides herself down onto it. Once he is comfortably inside her she wraps her legs tightly around his midriff, then locks her feet across his buttocks.

With the woman clinging to his shoulders, the man stands up very slowly, being careful to support her back and keep his balance until they are in an upright position (he should protect his back at moments of strain by bending his legs and keeping the woman close to his body). Locking his legs rigid and clutching her buttocks, the man swings her against him in short, sharp bursts.

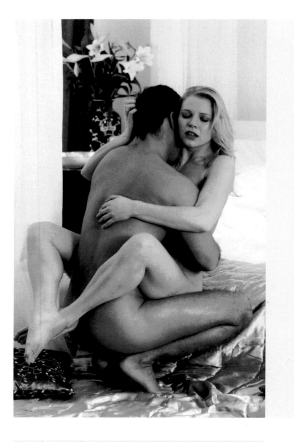

DIFFICULTY	🌸 🌸 🌸 🌼
TYPE	deep, intense, fast

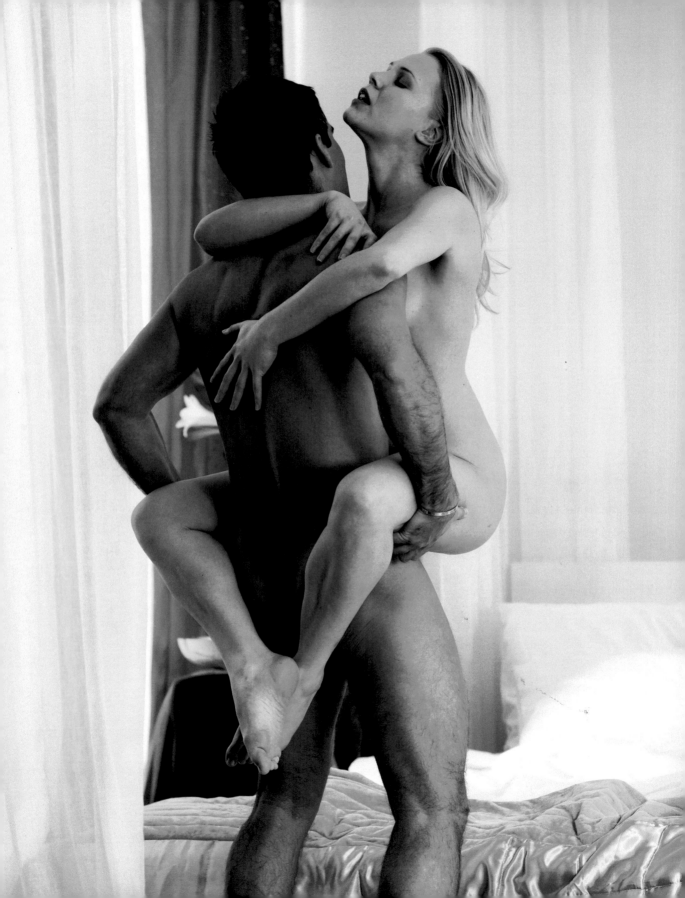

Driving the Peg

*'Whilst she is thus suspended, the man insinuates his pin into
her vulva, and the woman is then as if hanging on a peg.'*
Perfumed Garden

This position from the *Perfumed Garden* is a variation on Suspended Congress (page 112). Whilst motionless in this pose and confident of her lover's strength, the woman can lean back at arm's length, gripping the man's shoulders or arms, and being sure to maintain a tight grip with her legs around his midriff. He should make sure that he has one leg in front of the other to aid his balance. Although this posture does not allow the man to thrust deeply, this display of complete abandon by the woman is a visual feast for him and she will enjoy the acrobatics. Once they have tired of frolicking, the man may wish to lower his lover onto a table or bed, or hold her against a wall in order to reach climax.

DIFFICULTY	🌸 🌸 🌸 🌸
TYPE	intense, fast

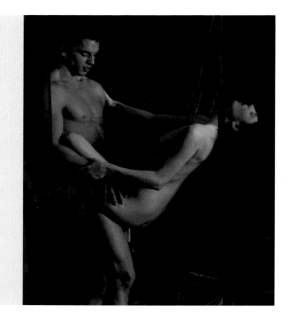

Getting Carried Away

Standing positions allow more mobility and give us a chance to make full use of our surroundings. Why not try moving from room to room (maintaining penetration if you can) and explore how different parts of furniture could act as props to your sexual drama.

For the man: lie your lover on the kitchen table and feast on her yoni or let yourself drop backwards onto the sofa so that she can take control. You could even try walking up the stairs. There is no end to the possible variations!

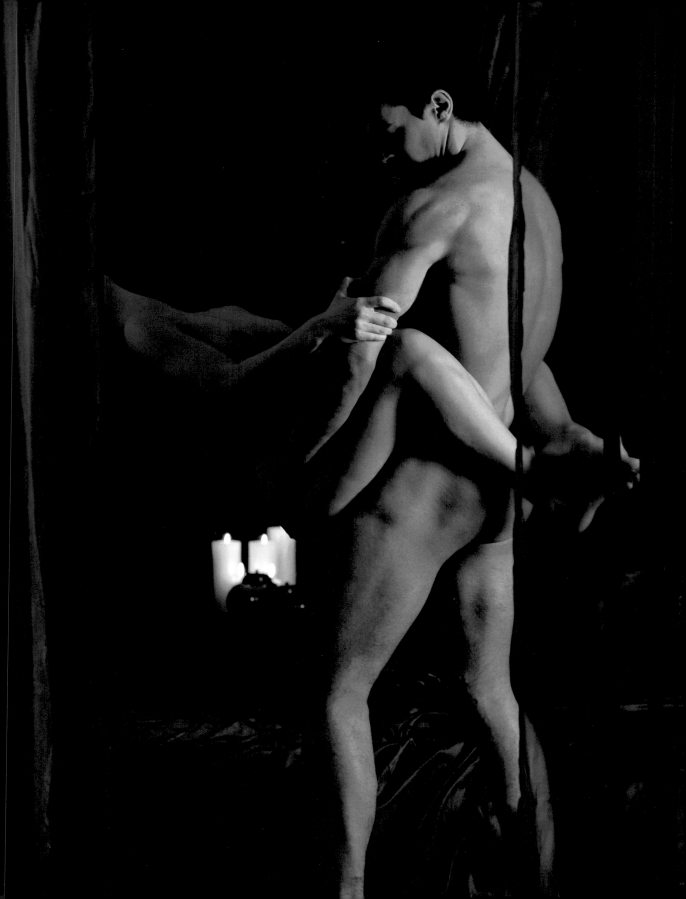

The Lotus

'She is called Padmini, or Lotus-woman. Her face is pleasing as the full moon; her body is soft as the mustard-flower; her skin is fine, tender and fair as the yellow lotus. Her eyes are bright and beautiful as the orbs of the fawn, well-cut, and with reddish corners. Her bosom is hard, full and high; her neck is goodly shaped as the conch-shell. Her yoni resembles the open lotus-bud, and her love-seed is perfumed like the lily which has newly burst.'

Ananga Ranga

The Lotus is a classic sitting pose from yoga and is greatly revered as a position for meditation and stillness. The lovers sit facing one another on a bed or rug, gazing at each other and feasting their eyes on their naked bodies to build up excitement.

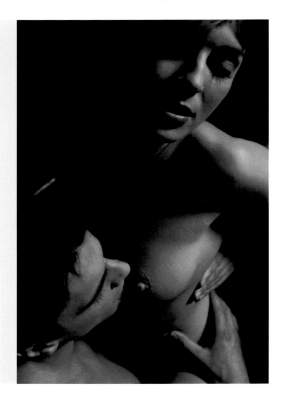

The man sits with his legs in a loose lotus position, displaying his penis and slowly playing with himself. When the time is right, the woman moves towards her lover and sits astride him, wrapping her arms and legs around his back.

This embrace binds the lovers together in a warm cocoon, and time should be taken to enjoy this feeling of unity. Let your hands roam and explore each other's skin, whilst gently nuzzling and kissing. To heighten arousal, the woman may gently brush her vagina against his penis assisted by the man supporting her buttocks.

DIFFICULTY	🌸 🌸 🌸 🌸
TYPE	gentle, slow

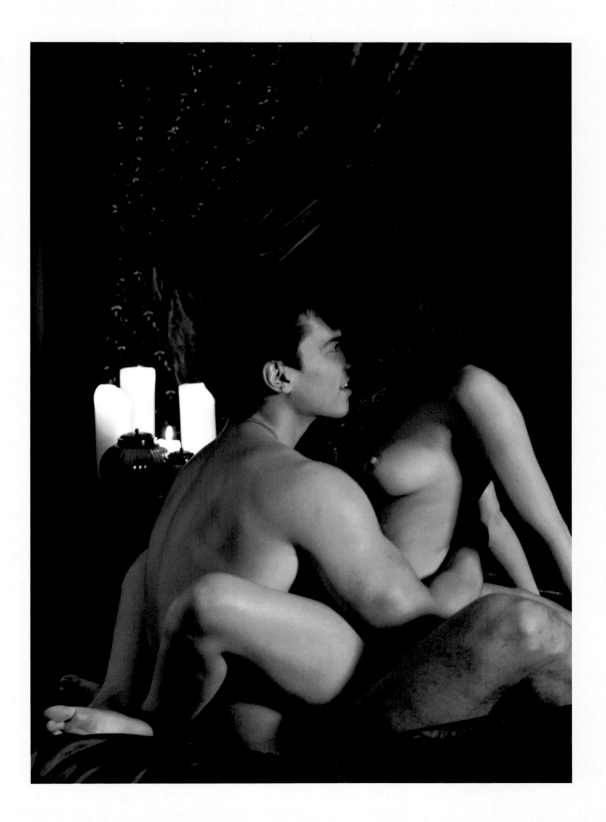

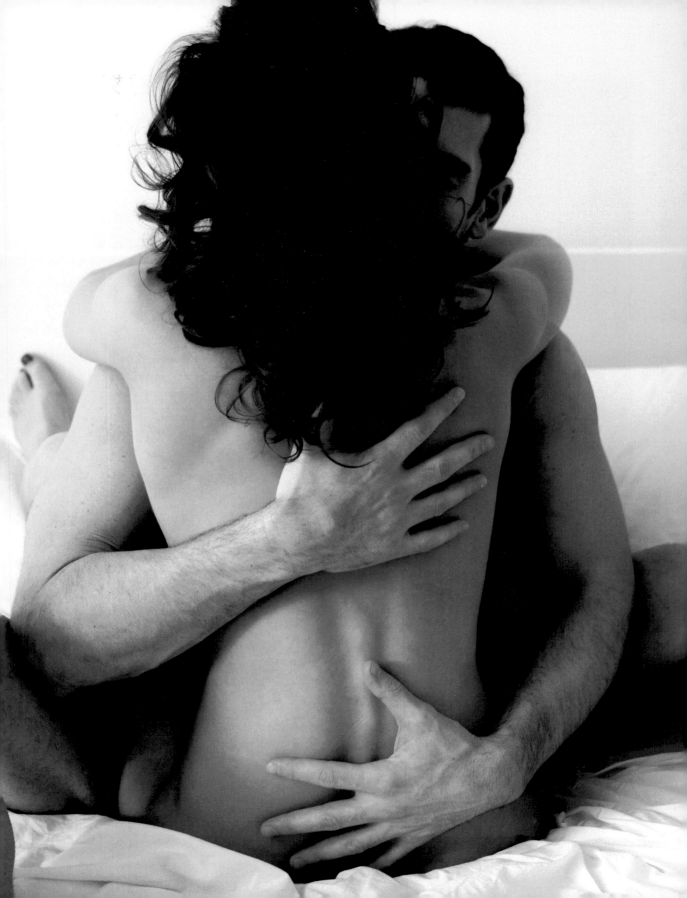

Chakras

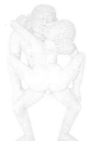

According to ancient Indian tradition, there are seven energy centres, or *chakras*, on the body which, when stimulated, can create a feeling of wholeness and wellbeing. These are often depicted as lotus petals and are located along the *Sushumna*, the central canal that corresponds to the spine, and are linked to each other by channels. The powerful creative force at the base of the spine is called *Kundalini* – Sanskrit for 'snake' – and is a double spiral of energy that can unlock sexual energy. According to Hindu tradition, when the *Kundalini* goddess is awakened, she uncoils and rises, unlocking the energies in each *chakra* as she travels towards the highest, at the crown. Once she has arrived at her destination, a person is said to have achieved enlightenment.

In Tantric sex, it is believed that high sexual arousal opens up the *chakras*, creating a sensation of oneness and ecstasy. Positions which encourage alignment of the *chakras* – where the spine is fully extended and the partners can breathe deeply together – and which allow the couple to look deeply into each other's eyes, are said to create an intense wave of rapture.

Imagining your lovemaking in terms of a sharing of these essential energies can help to increase the intimacy and warmth between you. As each *chakra* in your body is awakened by your increased sexual awareness and desire, you will begin to reach new heights of ecstasy never before experienced.

The Legraiser

UPAPAD

In the same posture as The Lotus, the woman leans back and places her hands on the floor behind her whilst the man supports her waist. She raises her left leg and, depending on her suppleness, places it over the man's right shoulder. In this position her movements will be limited so it is up to the man to gently roll his hips and sway forward and back to continue penetration. The important aspect of this position is close facial contact rather than vigorous sex. To avoid strain, the man should make sure his back is well supported. As a variation the woman can drop onto her elbows and place both legs over the man's shoulders to then slide against his groin.

DIFFICULTY	🌸 🌸 🌸
TYPE	gentle, slow

The Love Chamber

Don't forget that the secret to romance and great sex lies in creating the perfect mood and atmosphere and surrounding yourselves with sensual delights. Whether you choose to make love in the bedroom, living room, kitchen or bathroom (or all four), take time to create a relaxing and erotic backdrop.

Soften the lighting with candles, scent the air with burning oils or incense, lay fresh linen on the bed or perhaps construct a canopy above it. Scatter cushions on the floor, creating a nest for your lovemaking. Crack open a bottle of wine or champagne and prepare a platter of aphrodisiac foods that you can feed your lover. Put on a CD of your favourite sexy songs and close the door on any distracting sounds.

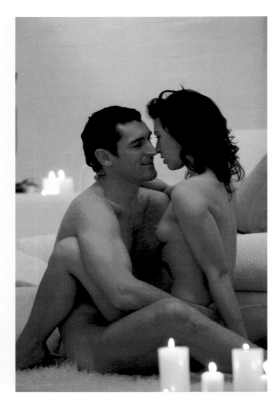

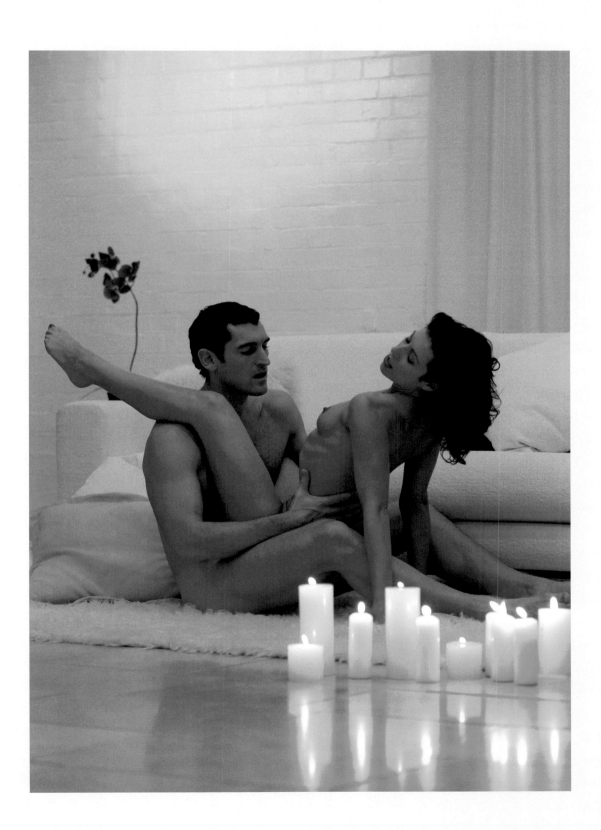

The See-Saw

YUGMAPAD

*'According to the poets, Yugmapad is that position in which
the husband sits with his legs wide apart, and, after insertion and
penetration, presses the thighs of his wife together.'*

Ananga Ranga

If following on from The Legraiser, the woman lowers her legs from the man's shoulders and places them tightly against his sides, tucking her feet in under him for support. The man opens his thighs just enough for the woman to slip down off his lap onto the cushions. This should be done slowly as it puts downward pressure on the penis and it is also easy to become disengaged. Clutching each other's wrists, both partners lean back carefully and begin to rock in a slow rhythm. Keeping her knees pressed together will maintain a tight squeeze on the

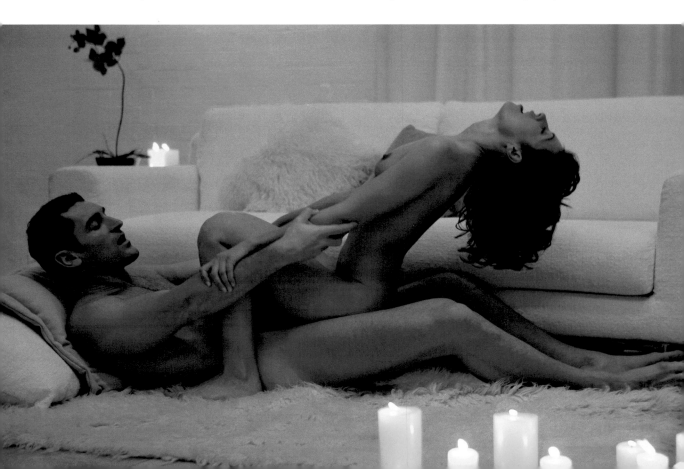

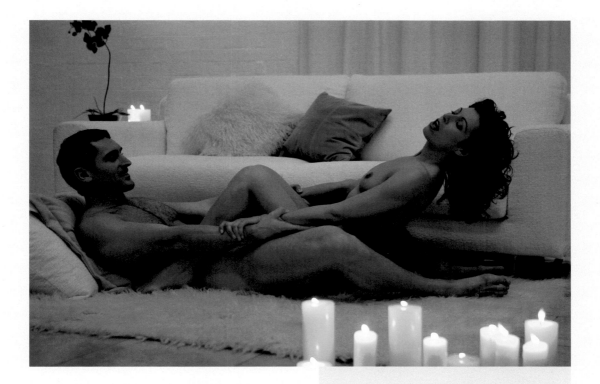

penis but it might be more pleasurable for her to open them so that both partners can see their genital union. Neither partner takes the lead in this position, which is one of mutual support and equal balance.

The posture can soon become a strain so it is important to have cushions placed behind each other for support and rest. Remember, very little movement is needed to feel full of each other's presence.

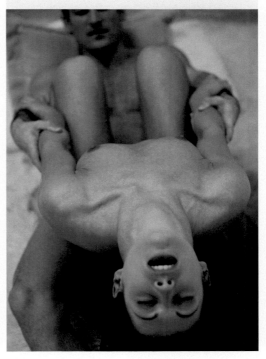

DIFFICULTY				
TYPE	gentle, slow			

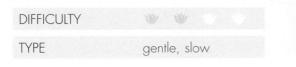

The Jointer

EL MODAKHELI

This is a good position to sink into once the couple has reached climax. The lovers recline right back onto cushions to rest from an intimate sex session. Mirroring each other, with legs intertwined, they lie apart but are still connected through the warmth and moistness of their genitals.

Feeling the energy of their recent lovemaking pulsating between them might heighten their arousal and they could easily slip into a gentle see-saw motion by reaching forward and grasping each other's arms before collapsing onto the cushions again.

With outstretched bodies their muscles can relax completely, allowing them to savour their intimacy in complete stillness and satisfaction. They may even wish to fall asleep like this.

DIFFICULTY	
TYPE	soft, gentle, slow

Sole Mates

Lying at opposite ends to each other, this position allows you to show your devotion to your lover by caressing their feet and slowly and methodically stimulating the reflex points. Take it in turns to apply pressure and mimic each move your lover makes so that everything that is received is also given.

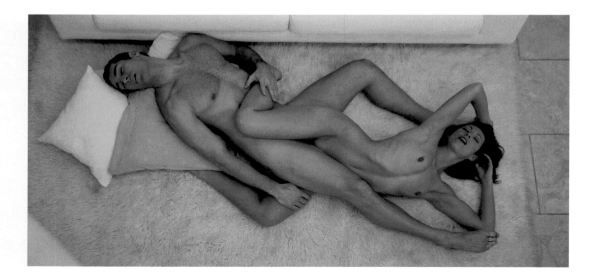

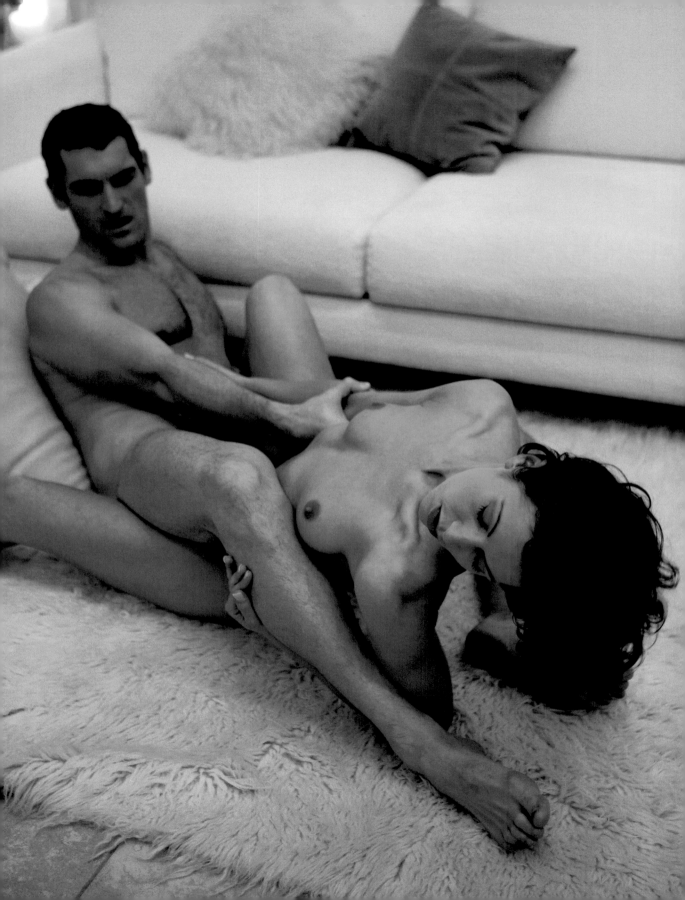

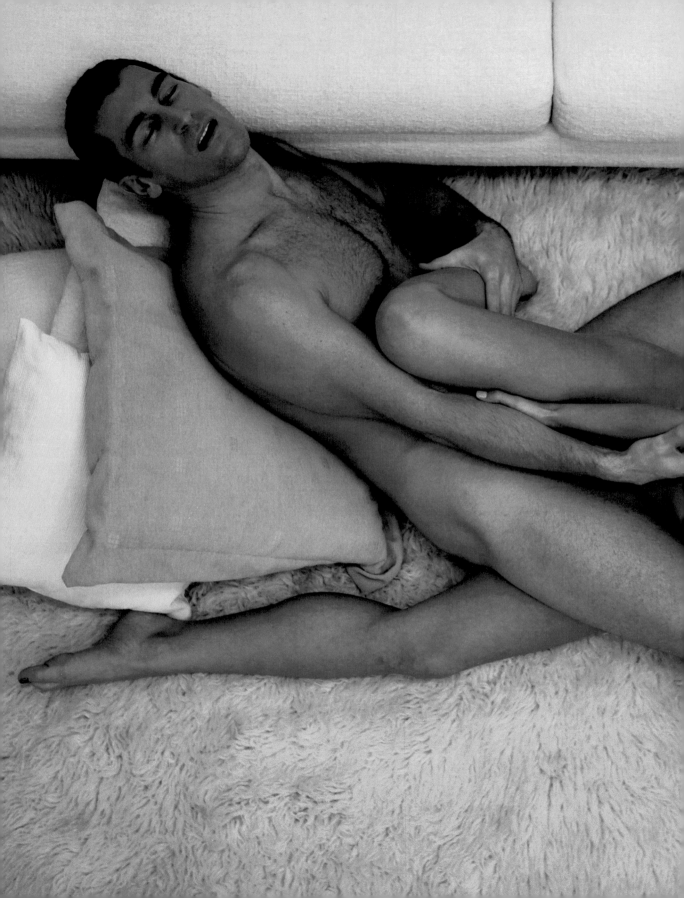

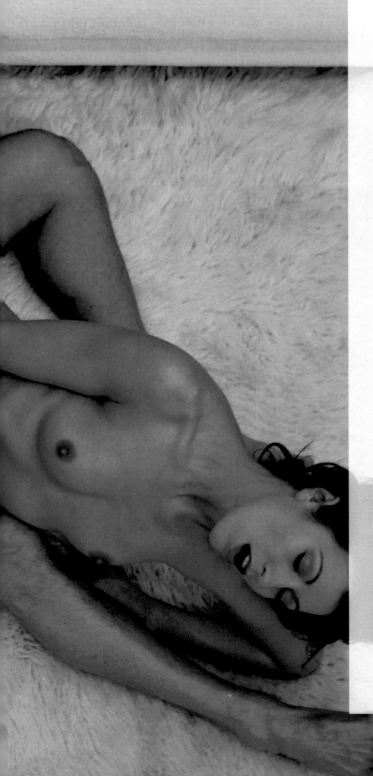

'When you observe the lips
of a woman to tremble and
get red, and her eyes to
become languishing, and
her sighs to become
quicker, know that she is
hot for coition; then get
between her thighs, so that
your member can enter
into her vagina.

If you follow my advice,
you will enjoy a pleasant
embrace, which will give
you the greatest
satisfaction, and leave you
with a delicious
remembrance.'

Perfumed Garden

The Tree Climber

*'When a woman...makes slightly the sounds of singing and cooing,
and wishes, as it were, to climb up him in order to have a kiss, it is
called an embrace like the "climbing of a tree".'*

Kama Sutra

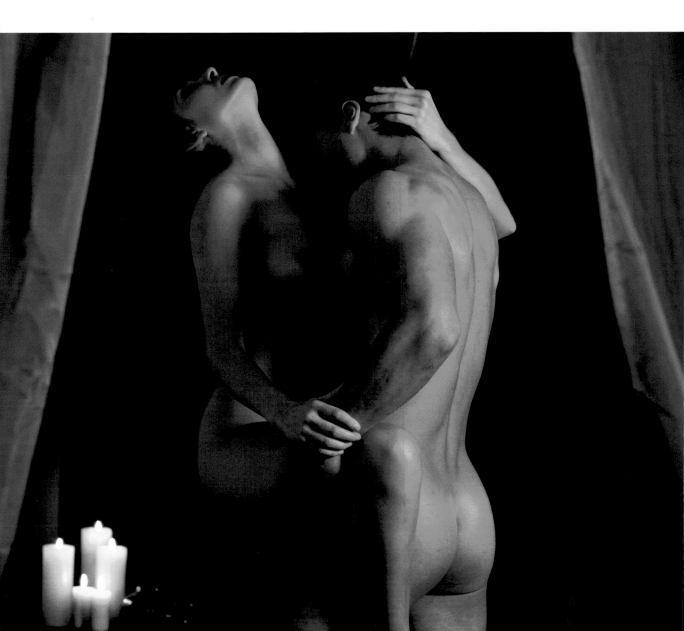

In this position, the lovers stand close together and, keeping their bodies tightly pressed, the woman places one arm around her lover's neck, and draws up her opposite leg around his thigh. Clinging tightly to him, she pulls his face towards hers and entices him to kiss her deeply and languorously. She arches her back, pushing out her breasts for him to enjoy. With his free hand, he can trace the contours of her body from her neck to her lifted foot. Placing her raised leg on a bed or chair and opening her thighs will help the man to penetrate her. The couple can gently grind their pelvic muscles but shouldn't get too carried away or they may lose their balance! For more vigorous grinding, both partners may find it easier when supported against a wall or the edge of a table.

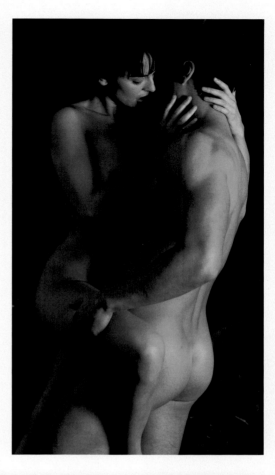

DIFFICULTY	
TYPE	gentle, slow

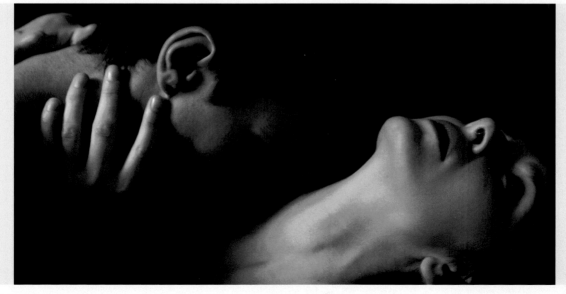

Suspended Congress

AVALAMBITAKA

According to the *Kama Sutra*, this position is described as 'Chitra' or amusing, since it is usually adopted in a jovial mood. It depends to some extent on the strength and agility of the man. He leans against a wall or table and the woman embraces him by encircling his neck with her hands and, clasping his thighs with hers, she places her feet against the wall or table. The man supports her by placing his hands on her buttocks or at the base of her spine. As the intensity rises, she can use the table for leverage to swing from side to side or backwards and forwards, as she rides her man to climax. Alternatively, he can turn her around and place her on the table so that he can thrust into her with greater vigour or let her reach climax by giving her oral sex.

DIFFICULTY	🪷 🪷 🪷 🪷
TYPE	deep, fast

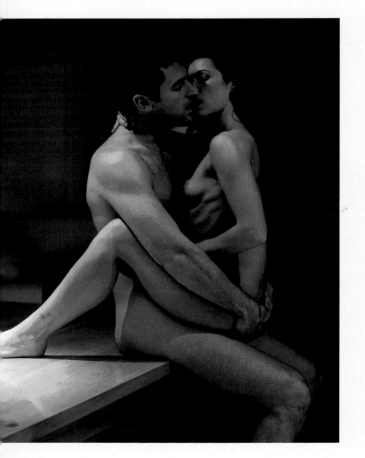

Limbering Up

Before trying some of the more demanding sexual positions, why not limber up with a few basic yoga exercises? Yoga is an integrated system of education for the body, mind and spirit and was part of daily life in India at the time the *Kama Sutra* was written.

Yoga is a great way of promoting health and wellbeing. Not only will it relax you and take away the stresses of the day, with practice, it will also help you to contort your body into sexual positions you had never even dreamt of!

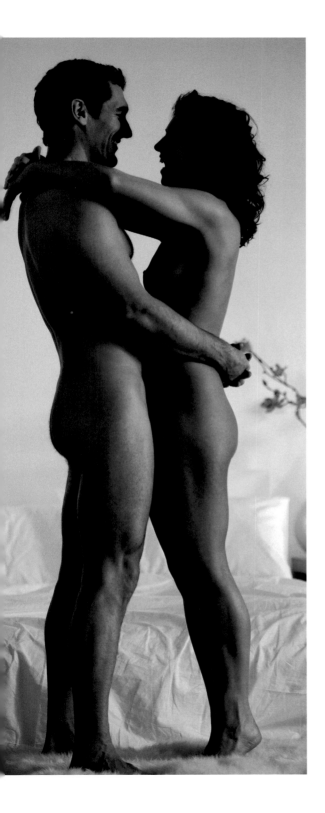

Humour in Sex

Sex doesn't always have to feel serious. Laughter and fun are essential ingredients to lovemaking and you will undoubtedly spice up your love life with a good dose of humour. It is also a great way to lose your inhibitions.

The *Kama Sutra* stresses the importance of learning the arts of 'magical sorcery' 'games', 'mimicry', 'riddles', 'puzzles' and 'dexterity in love-sport'. So be prepared to be playful; risk a new behaviour or activity; wrestle, pinch, tickle, or chase each other around the house.

You could invent your own love games: Make up a raunchy list of things to do to each other, assigning a number to each activity, then take it in turns to throw a dice to determine what delights you must deliver. Dress up, play naked games or use glow-in-the-dark body paint to write sexy messages on each other's bodies. Sitting opposite each other on a bed or carpet, the man can use his erect penis to catapult grapes or other edible morsels, with much precision and practice, into his lover's mouth! Above all, have fun!

The Hanging Bow

KIRTI-UTTHITA-BANDHA

'The Naisargiki-priti, or love-tie, is that natural affection by which husband and wife cleave to each other like the links of an iron chain. It is a friendship amongst the good of both sexes.'

Ananga Ranga

This position is perhaps more suited to yoga practitioners, as the woman needs to be supple and agile. It is a particularly rewarding position for the woman, as the headstand or handstand is one of the most powerful of yoga asanas (or postures), producing both mental and physical wellbeing.

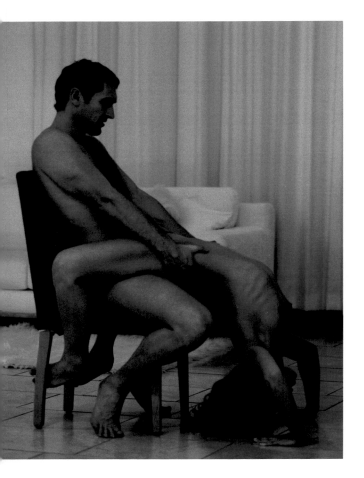

The man grips her hips firmly and leans back slightly, being sure to keep his balance. Letting go of his neck and clutching his forearms, the woman gradually lowers herself backwards until she is able to let go and place her hands on the ground in what appears as a handstand.

This posture completely changes the position of penetration, shortening the vagina and pressing the penis down, and may be easier for the man after climax. This pose demonstrates complete trust in each other's mobility and allows the body's natural energy to flow between the lovers. You can also experiment with this position by trying it with the man seated in a chair.

DIFFICULTY	🪷 🪷 🪷 🪷
TYPE	soft, intense

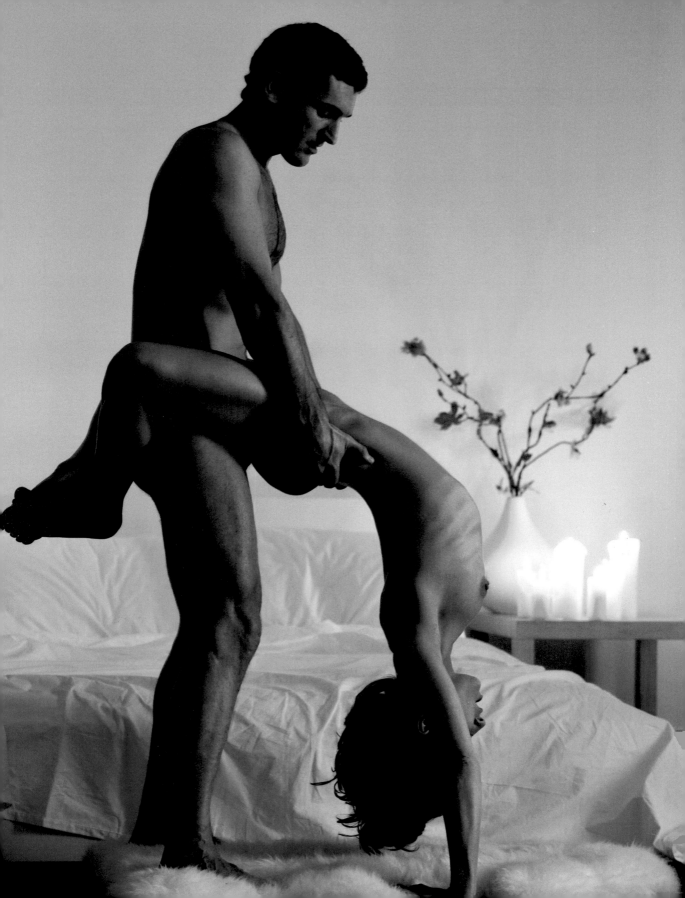

The Pair of Tongs

'When the woman holds the lingam in her yoni, draws it in, presses it, and keeps it thus in her for a long time, it is called the "pair of tongs".'

Kama Sutra

This is a good position for deep, fast sex and the woman is in complete control. The sequence can begin with the man sitting on a sofa or chair, fully or partially clothed. The woman may like to undress him quickly, then slowly peel off her clothes in front of him, watching as he hardens and becomes fully aroused. Turning her back to him she spreads her legs wide and straddles him, fondling and stroking his erect penis until she decides to lower herself onto it.

Clenching her vaginal muscles on him she can bounce up and down at her own pace and rhythm, or lean back to vary the angle of penetration. Because she is so wide open it is easy for her to play with her clitoris in a break from thrusting. The view of her backside grinding as she enjoys her man is a real turn-on for him.

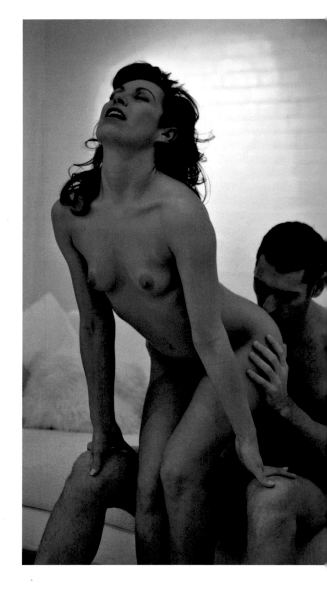

DIFFICULTY	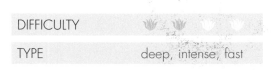
TYPE	deep, intense, fast

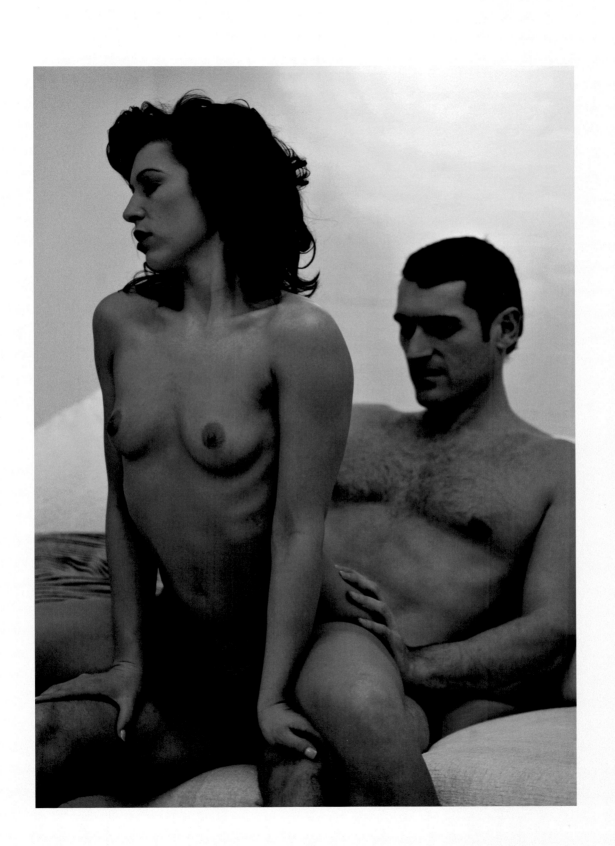

The Mounting of an Ass

GARDABHA

'At this time everything that is ordinarily done on the bosom should be done on the back. In the same way can be carried on the congress of a dog, the forcible mounting of an ass, the jump of a tiger, and the rubbing of a boar. And in all these cases the characteristics of these different animals should be manifested by acting like them.'

Kama Sutra

From The Pair of Tongs, the man opens his legs allowing the woman to place herself between his thighs and bring her knees together. This position gives intense pleasure to both partners, as it allows them to explore a variety of depths and angles so that all parts of the penis and vagina are stimulated. As she shifts from the last position to this one, the woman might like to play with the base of her lover's penis or fondle his testicles to help maintain his erection. The man leans forward and places his hands on her hips or reaches around to clasp her breasts or rub her clitoris. Bending her legs and holding onto his knees, the woman moves up and down on him in short, sharp bursts or with circular movements of her hips to stir him within her. She can change the angle of his penis by straightening her legs or squatting down further to find out just what feels best for her and for him.

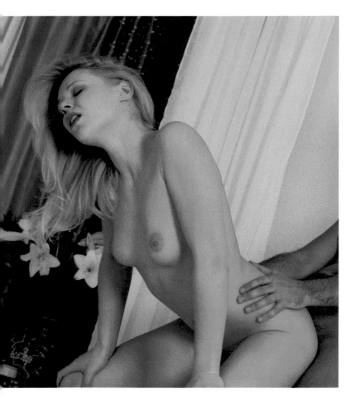

DIFFICULTY	🌸 🌸 ⚪ ⚪
TYPE	deep, intense, fast

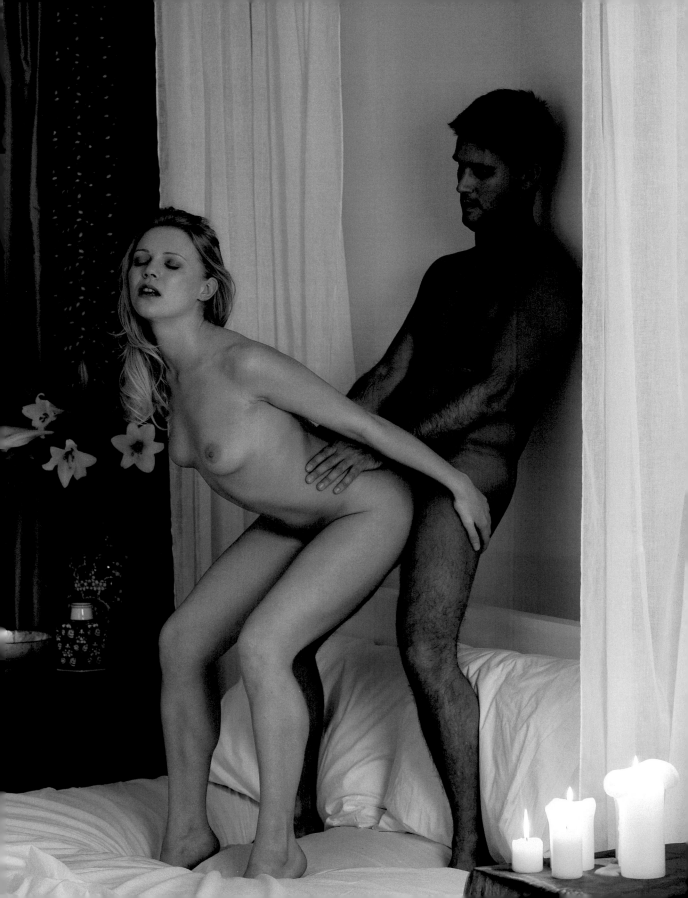

The Archer

The man gets down on bended knee, assuming an archer's stance (ready to shoot his Cupid's arrow!). At the same time, and maintaining a tight contact between them, the woman also drops onto her knees, preferably in front of a bed or sofa for her to lean against. The man pushes his raised leg between her thighs, thus forcing her to raise her right leg as well. He can kiss the nape of her neck and massage her back and shoulders.

Reaching down between her legs, she takes his penis in the palm of her hand and presses it against her vulva, slowly coaxing the tip between her labia.

As the man starts to enter her he can lift her leg and rest it on his bended knee to pierce her more deeply with his arrow.

DIFFICULTY	
TYPE	deep, slow

Alfresco Sex

Having sex outdoors can be really exciting as it provides a complete change of scenery and takes you away from distractions at home. There is also the added titillation of possibly being discovered. On a dirty weekend, try a shady wood, a moonlit beach or the centuries old tradition of a 'roll in the hay'.

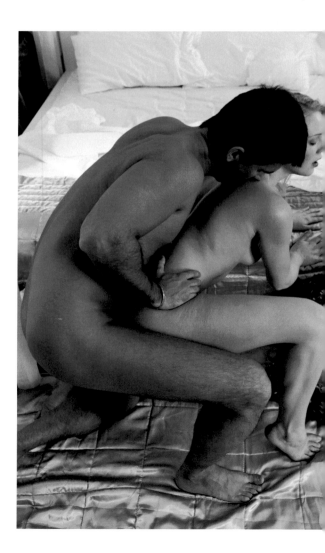

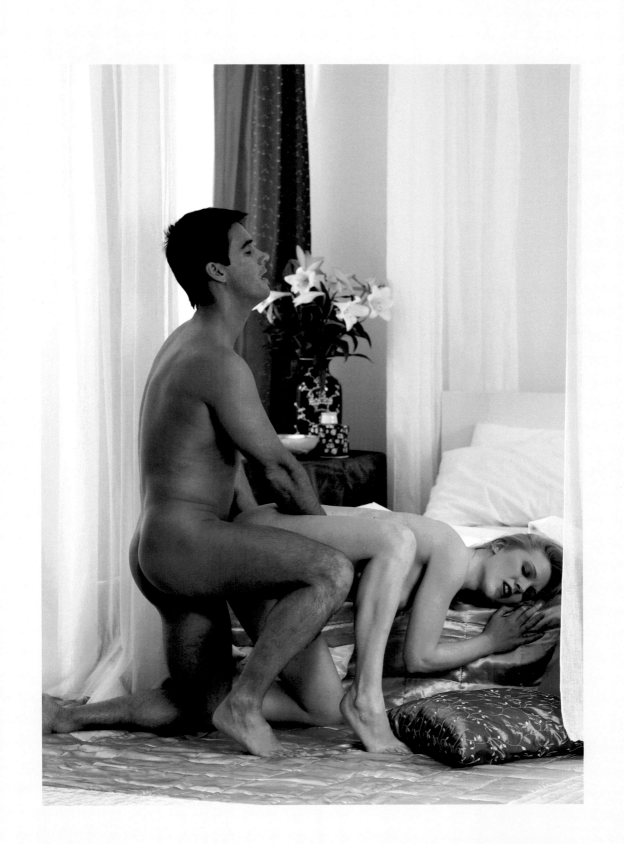

The Cats

In this pose, the man is completely in control, like a randy tom-cat overpowering his submissive feline. To get fully in touch with their bestial instincts, the couple may wish to perform this adventurous position outdoors.

The woman leans forward, supporting her weight on the bed or, if outside, perhaps on a garden bench. The man stands up slowly, while holding tightly onto the top of her thighs. To assist his movement and keep a firm hold, she should clamp her legs around his back. Locking his fingers together against her stomach to support her lower back, the man enters her slowly and, depending on the height of the bed, may need to bend his knees to find the best angle for his enjoyment. As this position allows very deep penetration, it can be extremely satisfying for both partners, but as the woman has no control, the man should take care not to get too carried away and should gauge her pleasure by the sounds that she makes.

DIFFICULTY	🌷 🌷 🌷 🌷
TYPE	deep, intense, fast

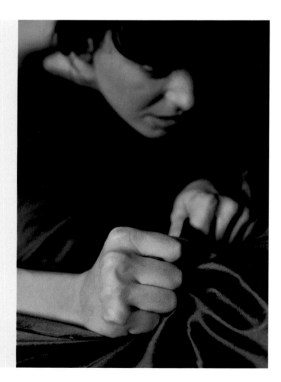

Sexy Sounds

The *Kama Sutra* talks about the amorous sounds of pleasure during sex: 'When a man indulges in kissing and in other modes of arousing her passion, the woman should respond in the same way and utter cries of joy and other shrieks.' This can be a great way to compliment your lover and let them know that you are really aroused. As well as being a sexy turn-on for your lover, a deep moan can awaken all your *chakras* when it resounds through your body.

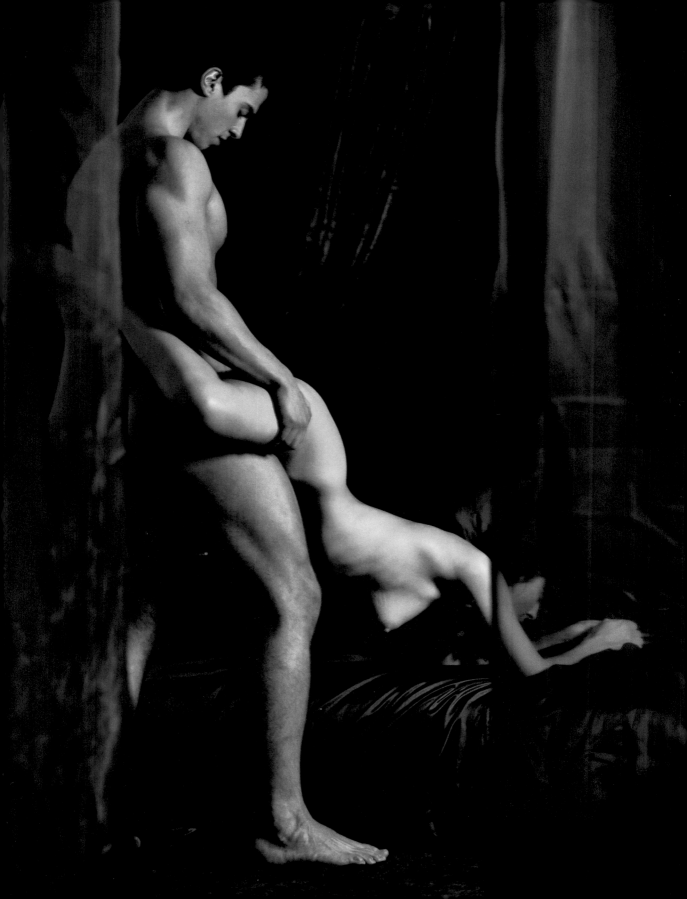

The Camel's Hump

AL SANAM AL NAKAH

'If the man withdraws while the woman is still bending down, the vagina emits a sound like the bleating of a calf, and for that reason women object to the posture!'
Perfumed Garden

With her feet slightly apart, the woman bends forward and rests her elbows on a low sofa or bed. Standing behind her, the man rubs the tip of his penis against her exposed labia pushing it half way in, then retrieving it, tantalising and toying with her. With her vagina exposed to him so wantonly, he may be tempted to start thrusting straight away but circling or 'churning' his penis within her first is a gentler approach before the more vigorous motions that usually accompany this position. As well as varying the rhythm and depth of penetration as much as possible, it is particularly pleasurable if he uses shallow thrusts at the entrance to her vagina. Watching himself entering and withdrawing from the woman is an added thrill for him.

DIFFICULTY	🌸 🌸 🌸 ◗
TYPE	deep, intense, fast

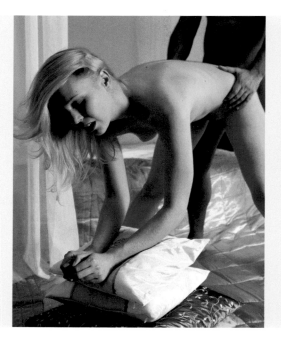 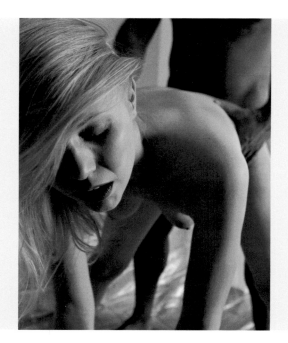

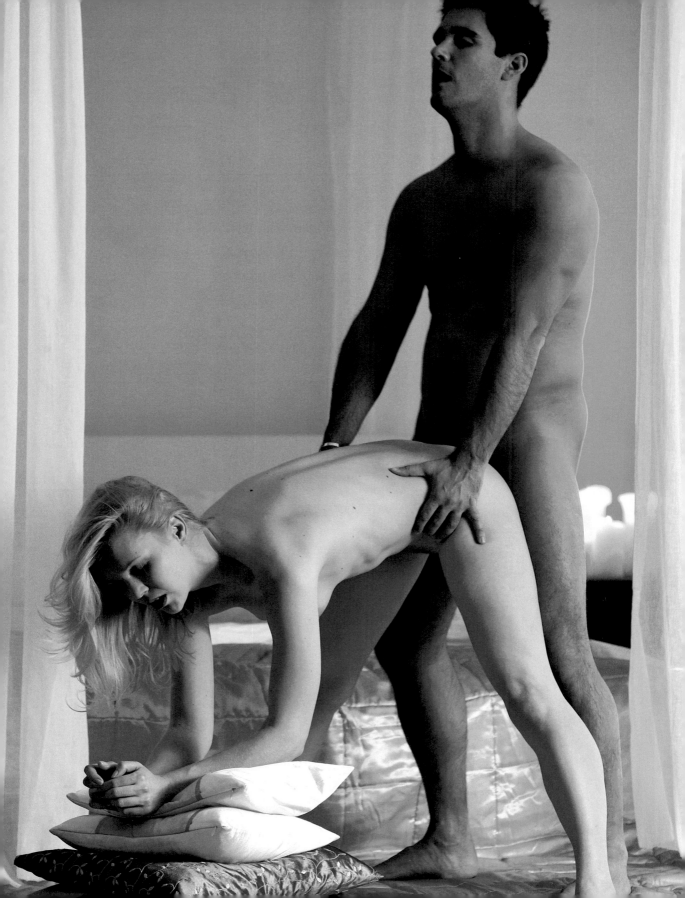

The Embrace of the Thighs

URUVAGUHANA

'She acts the man's part from the beginning. At such a time, with flowers in her hair hanging loose, and her smiles broken by hard breathings, she should press upon her lover's bosom with her own breasts, and lowering her head frequently, should do in return the same actions which he used to do before.'

Kama Sutra

This is a wonderfully intimate position where the woman entraps her man between her thighs in a strong clench. The man is seated on a firm comfortable chair, preferably with a tall back. The woman tells him to close his eyes and not to move as she kneels and parts his legs, stimulating him alternately with her mouth and hands until he is erect. Then, facing him, she straddles his thighs and gently lowers herself onto his penis. From this position she can determine her own rhythm – up and down, rocking to and fro, or grinding in a circular motion. She may like to squeeze his shoulders with each motion or massage his neck and head, whilst at the same time he is able to kiss and suck her breasts and nipples. She could try blindfolding him so that each movement she makes comes as a great surprise!

DIFFICULTY

TYPE — deep, intense

The Love Bite

The *Kama Sutra* devotes an entire chapter to biting, suggesting that all the places that can be kissed are also the places that can be bitten. Names such as 'the broken cloud' and 'the coral and the jewel' were given to these naughty nibbles.

Biting your lover on various parts of the body can add an extra sensation during sex and today, as in ancient times, lovers can enjoy the sight of bite marks inflicted on each other as a memento of their previous sexual pursuits.

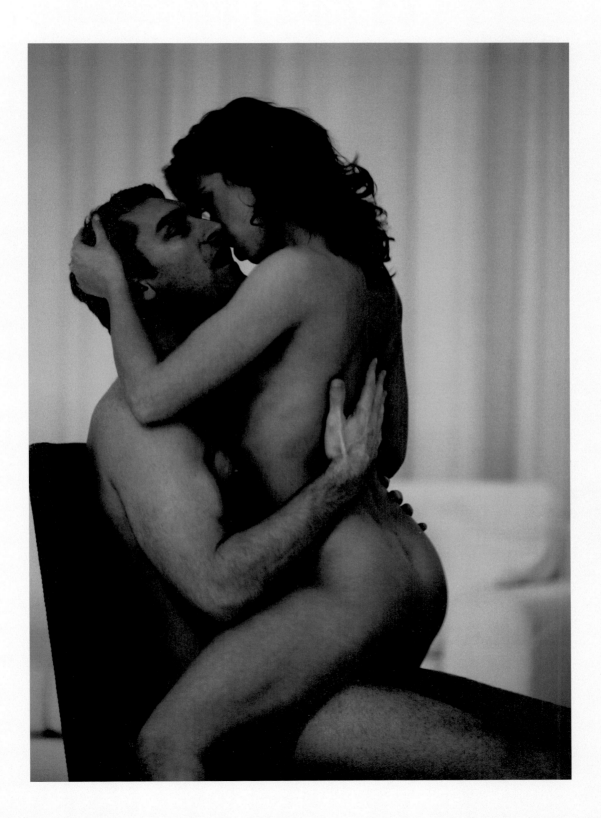

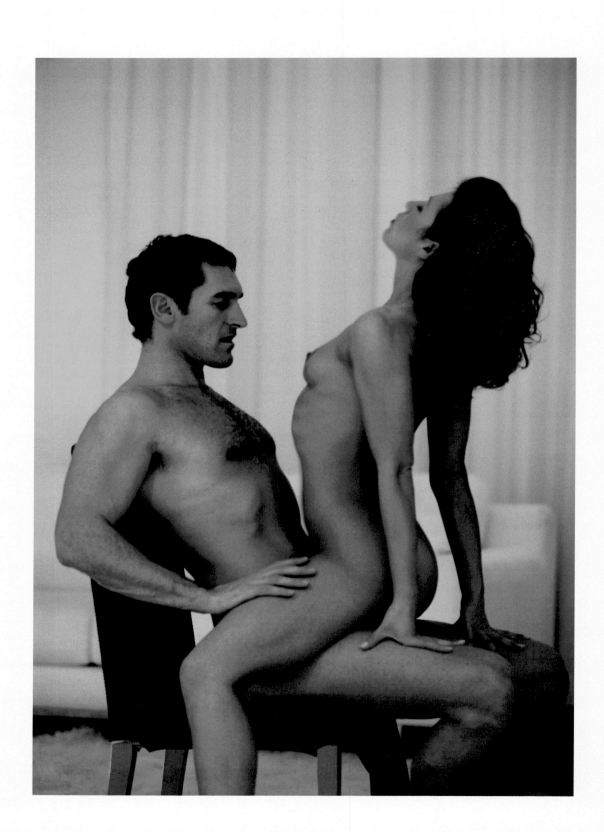

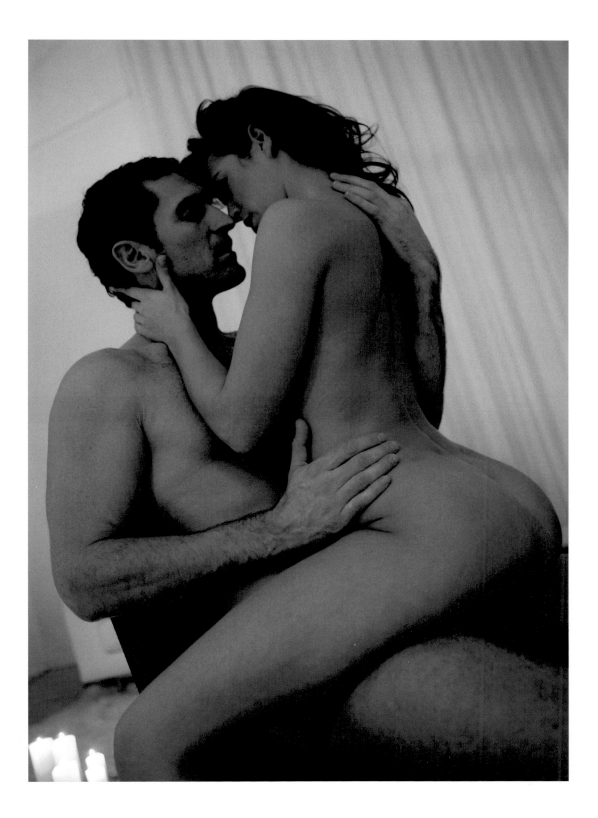

Pounding the Spot

DOK EL ARZ

This position can continue from The Embrace of the Thighs. Holding onto the man's neck, the woman arches her spine and throws back her head in an erotic display that shows she is full of desire and ready to yield to her burning passion. She lifts her feet slightly, opening up to him, thus increasing the angle and depth of his penis within her.

The man grips her hips and slides her up and down on his penis in a pulsating rhythm. She will receive clitoral stimulation as she pounds against his pubic bone. By raising and lowering her legs alternately she will heighten his enjoyment with a slow rolling penis massage. To assist her he may hook his arms under her legs so that her knees are bent over his elbows. She can then support her weight by holding his knees and using them as a lever to push herself up and down on him.

DIFFICULTY	🌸 🌸 🌸 🤍
TYPE	deep, intense, fast

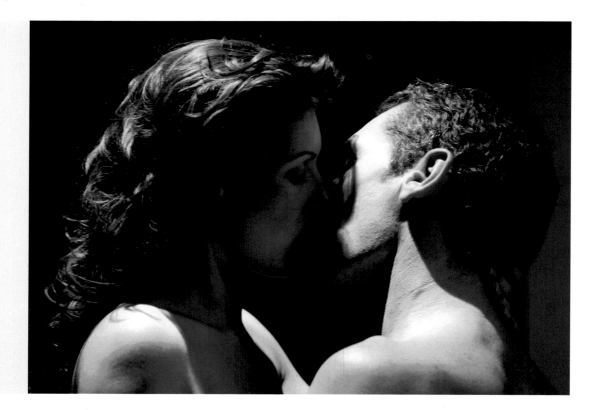

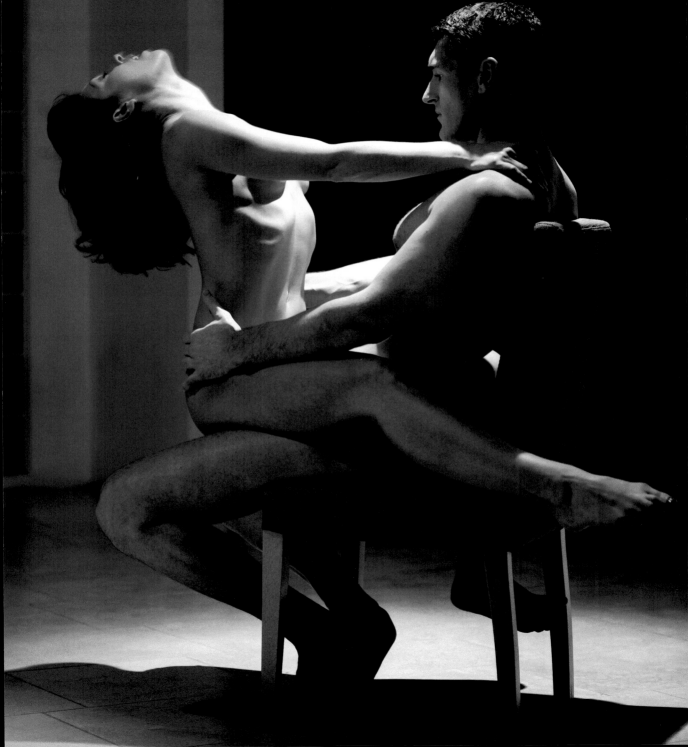

The Spinning of the Top

BHRAMARAKA

'When the woman is on top of the man, holding his lingam in her yoni, and she turns round like a wheel, it is called the 'top'. This is learnt by practice only.'

Kama Sutra

Continuing from Pounding the Spot, the man sits back on the chair and the woman, holding onto one of his shoulders, leans back slightly and passes one of her legs over his head so that she comes to sit sideways on his lap. This may take a little practice and might depend on the suppleness of the woman and the length of the man's penis. She turns again slowly and sits astride his legs, taking his penis deep inside her and using her vaginal muscles to grip and squeeze it tightly as she moves up and down.

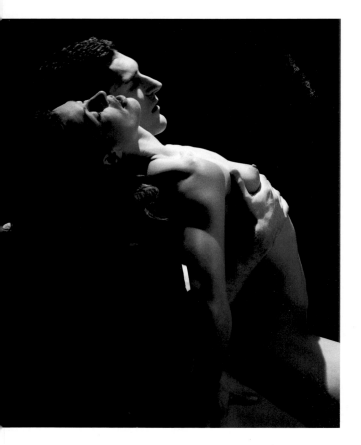

Holding onto a table will help to take some of the strain off her legs, and the man can assist by pushing her buttocks to and fro. Doing this position in front of a mirror is an added turn-on, as it introduces an element of voyeurism and the lovers will be able to watch their bodies in motion and their genitals moving together.

The woman can sustain pleasure by using her vaginal muscles to grip the penis inside her for as long as possible, as though 'milking' it, letting it slowly withdraw as it becomes flaccid. This is known as the 'mare's trick' and can be learnt through practice.

DIFFICULTY	🌸 🌸 🌸 🌼
TYPE	deep, fast

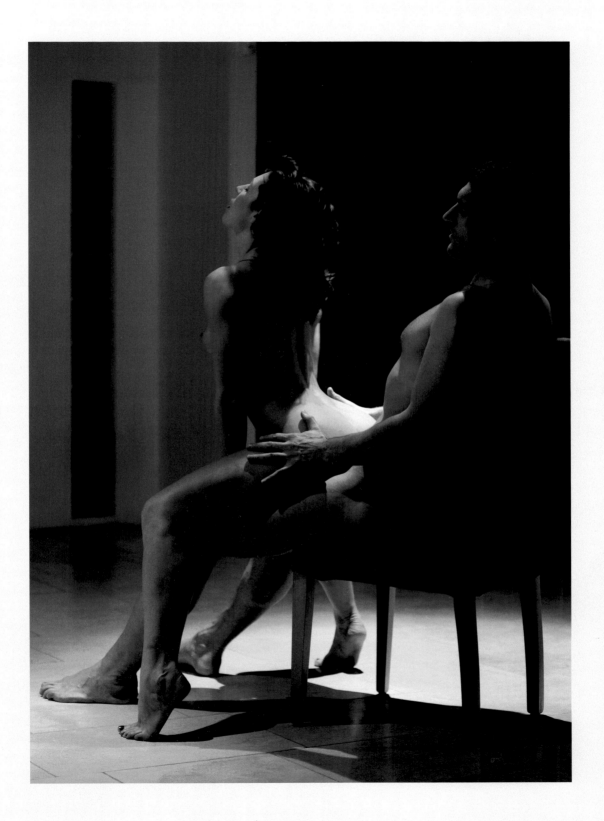

Woman on Top

'When a woman sees that her lover is fatigued by constant congress, she should lay him down upon his back, and give him assistance by acting his part. She may also do this to satisfy the curiosity of her lover, or her own desire of novelty.'

Kama Sutra

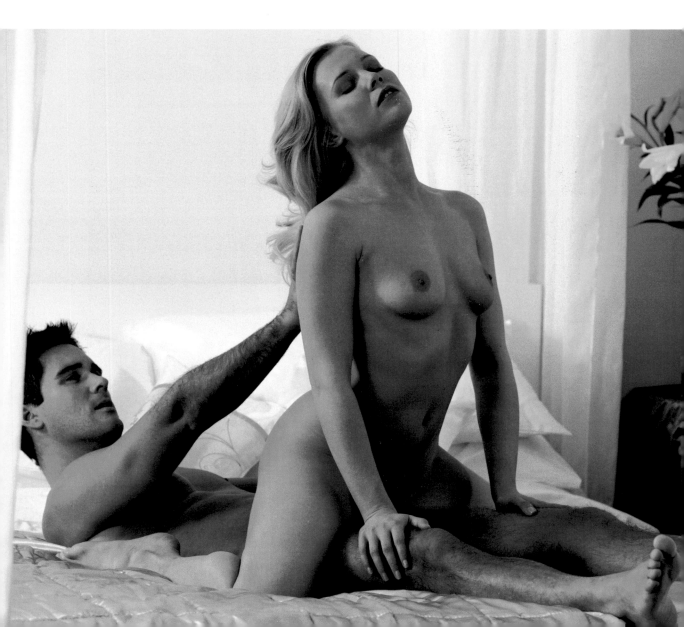

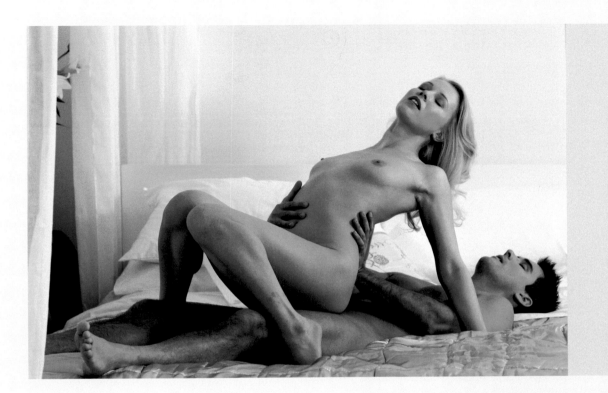

It is good to move into this position from a deliciously slow session of Kakila, or sixty-nine. When the couple is close to climax, the woman slides down the man's body and straddles him in a kneeling position.

Whilst holding onto his thighs, she plunges him deep inside her. The woman has all the control, and is free to grind and swivel her hips so that his penis touches her in all the right places. She can lean back far enough for the man to grasp her shoulders or if she prefers to sit up straight, he can knead her buttocks or bend his arms to reach and massage her feet, thus maintaining their bond. With the man supporting her back firmly, the woman can raise her knees and then gradually lean back with her arms outstretched

to the floor behind her. She should be careful not to put too much pressure on the man's abdomen and should lift herself up slightly by resting on the balls of her feet.

Clamping her knees together will increase the squeeze on his penis, and varying her angle slightly will cause it to rub against the upper wall of her vagina. The man clasps her sides and begins to glide her rhythmically up and down. He will need good upper body strength to maintain this for any length of time so the couple may wish to move on to an easier position quite soon.

DIFFICULTY	⚜ ⚜ ⚜ ⚜
TYPE	intense, fast or slow

Sporting of the Swan

'Being still full of the water of love, the wife must, therefore, place her husband supine upon the bed or carpet, mount upon his person, and satisfy her desires.'

Kama Sutra

For many women this is the best way to reach orgasm during sex, as she controls the rhythm and speed as well as the depth of penetration. It is also good for stimulation of the G-spot. Facing away from him, the woman squats over her lover and mounts his penis. Tucking her feet in close to his upper thighs and with her hands placed on his hips or knees, she rides her lover with vigorous thrusts.

The woman can try varying these thrusts, perhaps five shallow followed by one deep, and she can use her fingers to squeeze her labia onto his shaft. This position provides a very pleasing sight for the man as he can luxuriate whilst his lover abandons herself to her desires.

DIFFICULTY	🌸 🌸 🌸 🌸
TYPE	deep, intense, fast

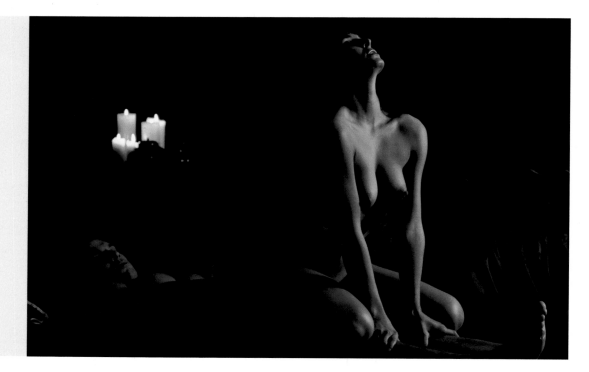

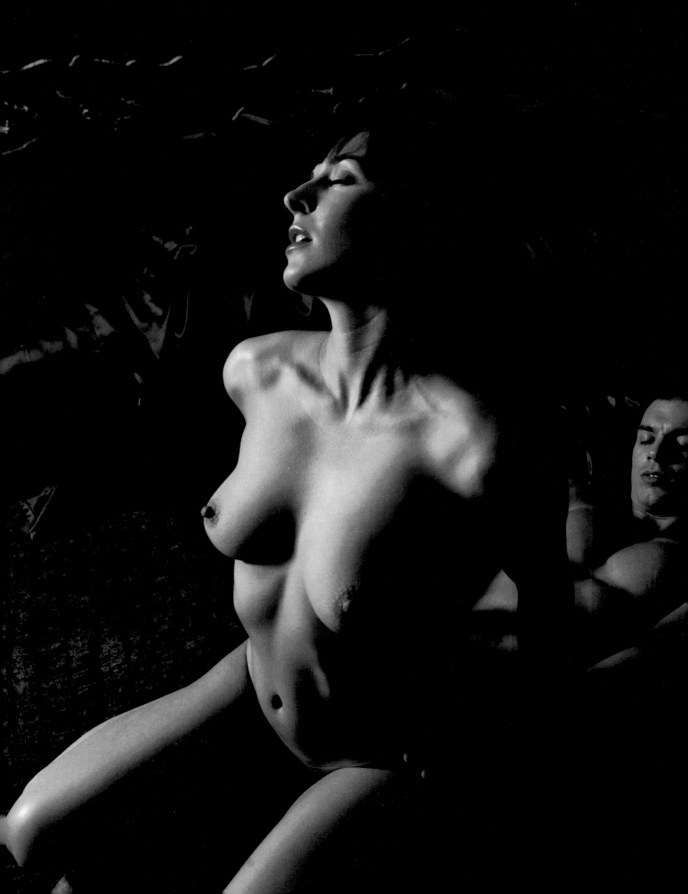

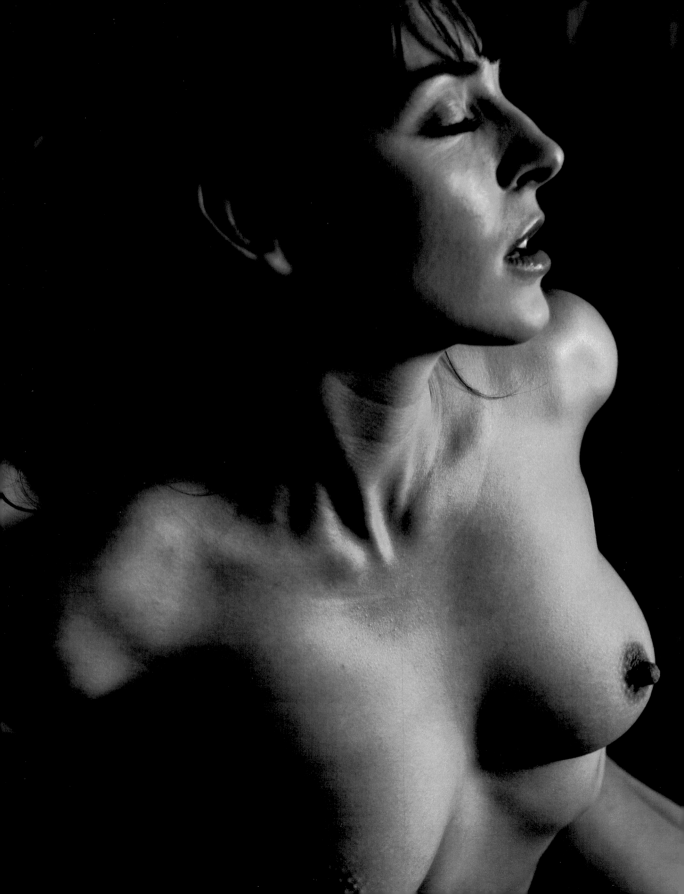

The G-spot

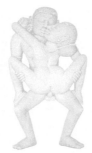

This elusive but famous organ in the vagina is named after Dr Ernst Gräfenberg, who apparently 'discovered' it in the 1950s, although clear mention of it is made in certain Indian texts dating as far back as the 11th century. The *Ananga Ranga* describes it thus:

'Moreover, in the yoni there is an artery called Saspanda, which when excited by the presence and energetic action of the linga, causes Kamasalila (the water of life) to flow. It is inside and towards the navel, and it is attached to certain roughnesses (thorns), which are peculiarly liable to induce the paroxysm when subjected to friction.'

It is not entirely certain whether all women have a G-spot, but many women reportedly get great satisfaction from its stimulation – in addition to clitoral or purely vaginal stimulation – so if you are comfortable exploring your own body, you can try to locate it. Insert a finger into your vagina and press against the front vaginal wall, about 5cm inside and near the base of the urethra. You should find a small area of spongy raised tissue about the size of a button. When you rub this, you may feel like you need to urinate but this sensation quickly passes and the area becomes erect and feels pleasurable to the touch.

Rear entry and woman-on-top positions are best for its stimulation. The orgasm you can achieve might be harder to obtain but is apparently deeper and more intense.

The Mutual View of the Buttocks

From a lying position, the man sits up with his legs slightly apart and leans back on his hands or against a bedstead. After a vigorous session of Sporting of the Swan and, with his penis still inside her, the woman draws her legs together between his and leans forward to place her palms upon the floor. This movement will delight the man by squeezing his penis. He keeps a firm hold on her by clenching his thighs on her buttocks, and in this pose they gently rock to and fro. The woman leans back and rests against his chest so that he can envelop her with his arms, stroking her breasts and massaging her abdomen. She will be hot from her exertions so he could blow gently on her back and shoulders to cool her down.

DIFFICULTY	🌸 🌸 🌸 🌸
TYPE	intense, slow

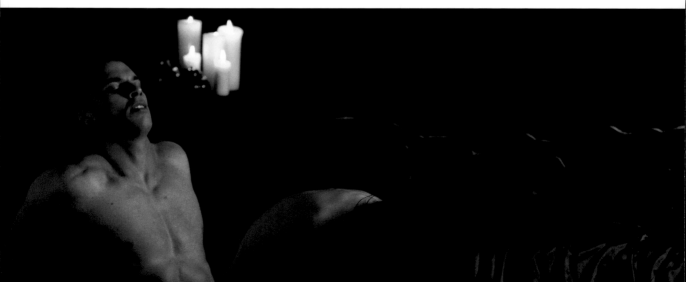

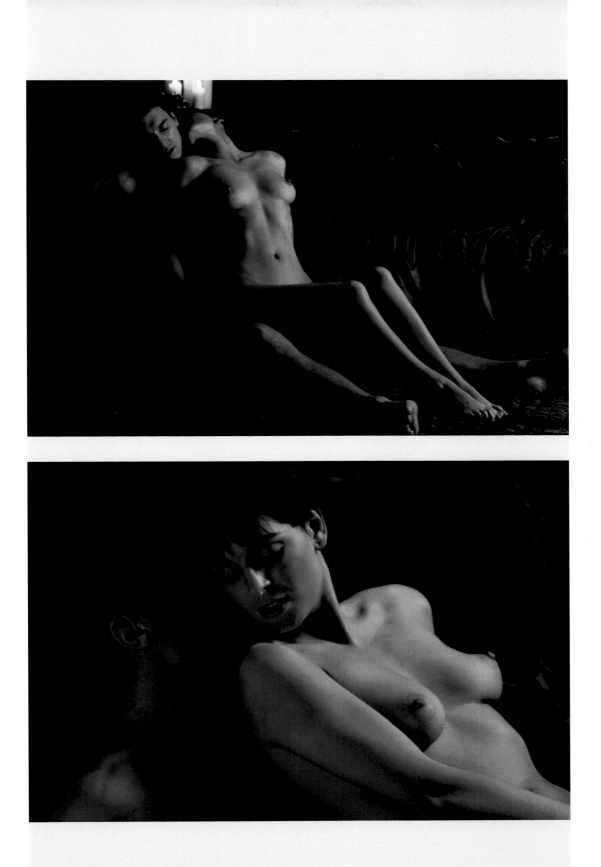

Milk and Water

KSHIRANIRAKA

'When a man and a woman are very much in love with each other and embrace each other as if they were entering into each other's bodies, either while the woman is sitting on the lap of the man, or in front of him, or on a bed, then it is called an embrace like a "mixture of milk and water".'

Kama Sutra

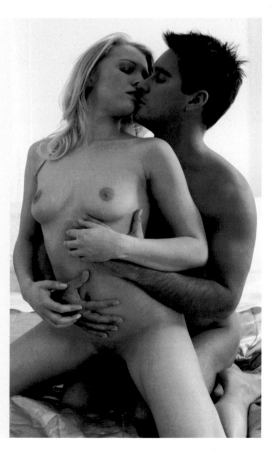

This position can begin with a simple loving embrace that builds up intimacy and warmth between the lovers. With plenty of comfy cushions or bedding beneath them, the man sits on his feet with the woman astride his lap, facing away from him. He envelops her in his arms and she invites him to play with her clitoris, guiding his fingers and showing him exactly what she wants. With his penis resting between her buttocks, she clenches her cheeks to squeeze and stimulate him. She will enjoy the sensation of him hardening beneath her. When she is moist and swollen with excitement she lifts herself up ever so slightly and lowers herself onto him. Cheek-to-cheek, they hold each other so tightly that they feel fused as one.

DIFFICULTY	🌸 🤍 🤍 🤍
TYPE	soft, gentle, slow

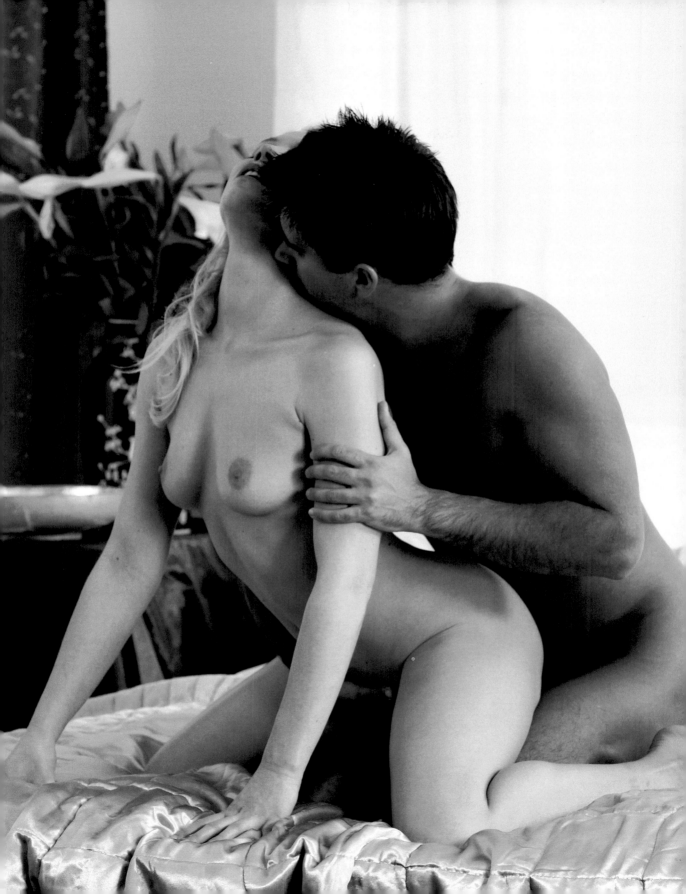

The Ram

EL KABACHI

'Such passionate actions and amorous gesticulations or movements, which arise on the spur of the moment, and during sexual intercourse, cannot be defined, and are irregular as dreams... a loving pair become blind with passion in the heat of congress, and go on with great impetuosity, paying not the least regard to excess.'

Kama Sutra

If moving on from Milk and Water, the man moves off his haunches, clasping her hips whilst maintaining penetration. The woman leans forward and drops onto her hands, arching her back and raising her head. Depending on preference, either the man or the woman can control the speed and rhythm of movement.

The man may remain still, while the woman moves as she likes – side to side, up and down, in and out – whatever she finds most pleasurable, or she may indicate that she would like him to move inside her while she steadies her body by gripping the side of the bed.

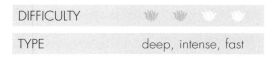

DIFFICULTY	🌸 🌸 🌸 🌸
TYPE	deep, intense, fast

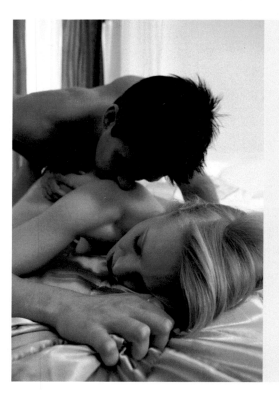

Mirrored Image

For the woman: Without the intimacy of face-to-face contact, the woman might like to place a hand mirror beneath her, angling it so that she can enjoy watching the man sliding in and out of her.

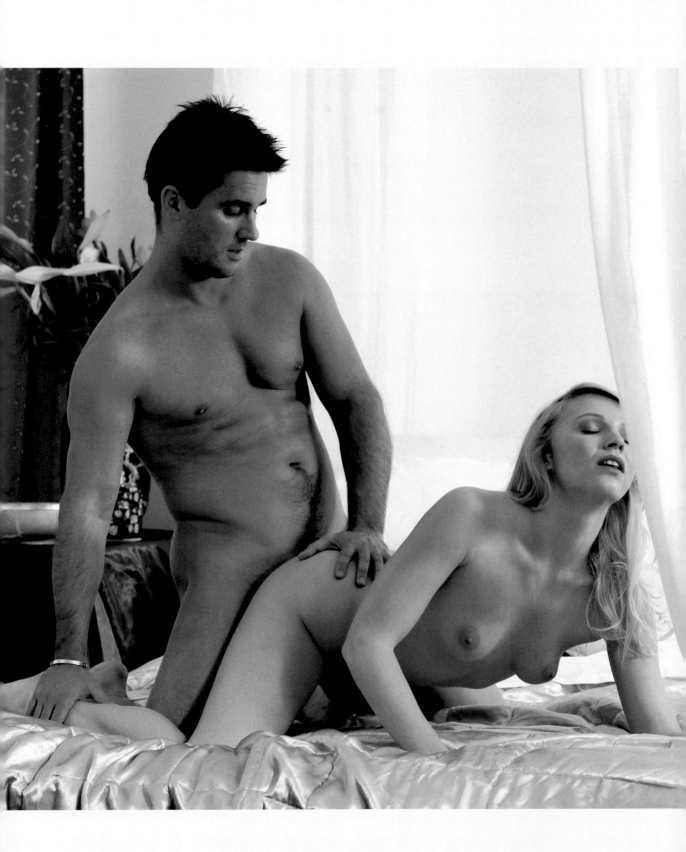

Coition from Behind

NIK EL KOHOUL

*'The man approaches from behind, stretches himself on her
back and inserts his tool while the woman twines her arms round
the man's elbows. This is the easiest of all methods.'*

Perfumed Garden

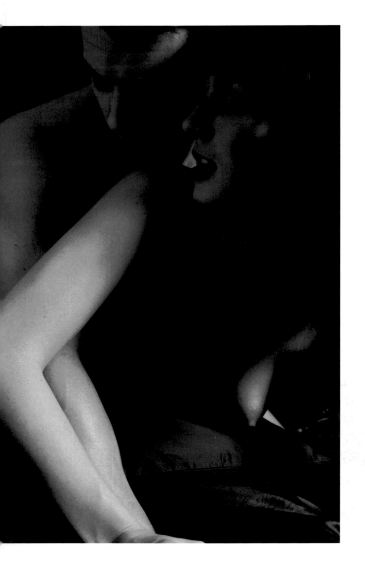

Although many Indian writers on eroticism revered front-entry positions, they recognized that these did not allow full stimulation of the clitoris. To overcome this problem, they recommended rubbing the clitoris manually or with the penis. Rear-entry positions like this one, though, don't present such a problem, as the angle of penetration naturally affords a fuller stimulation of the clitoris. A small amount of pressure on her mons pubis (or pubic mound) whilst he is mounting her is likely to send her into paroxysms of pleasure. With the aid of cushions propped beneath her, her vulva is displayed more prominently, allowing her lover to maintain comfortable penetration. Dropping with her, he can support himself with his arms either side of her, or by pressing down on her buttocks with both hands as he thrusts. Rubbing against the cushions as he does this may be sufficient for her to reach orgasm.

DIFFICULTY		
TYPE	deep, intense, fast	

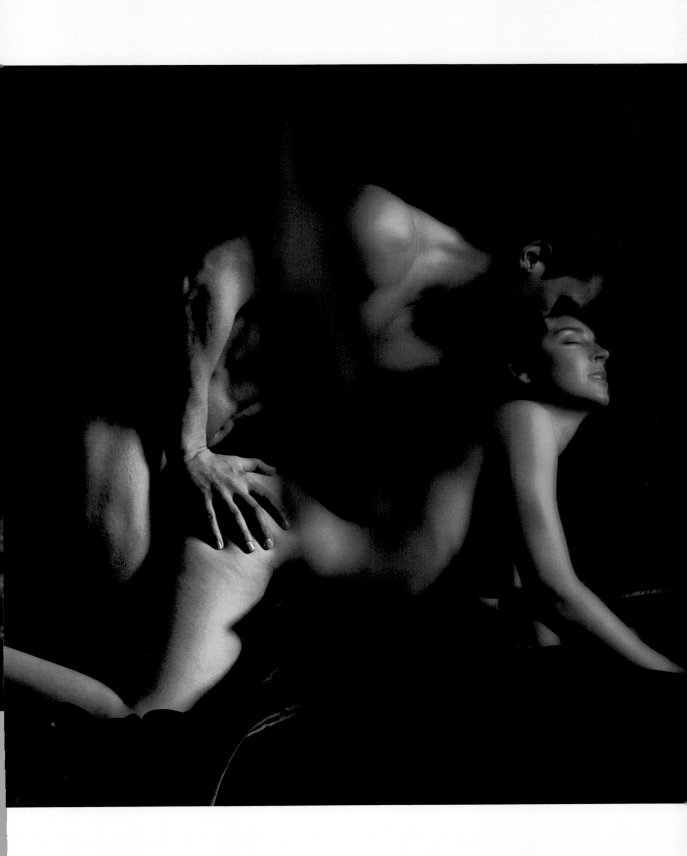

The Side Clasp

After orgasm in Coition from Behind, the man lies spent across his lover's back, his deep breaths resonating in her ears. They clasp hands and the man moves his legs either side of his lover's so that he is encasing her in a loving hold. When they are rested and ready, the couple roll to one side, and the woman then manoeuvres herself so that she is lying on her back at right angles to him. It may be possible to maintain penetration throughout but it's not essential as the main aim of this pose is for the couple to relax and have close eye contact after a tiring session. The man's hands are free to stroke his lover's body or, if desired after time, to start arousing her again.

DIFFICULTY	🪷 🪷 🪷 🪷
TYPE	soft, gentle

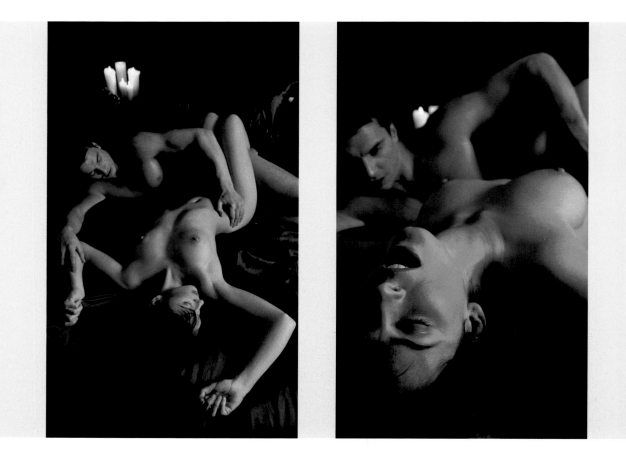

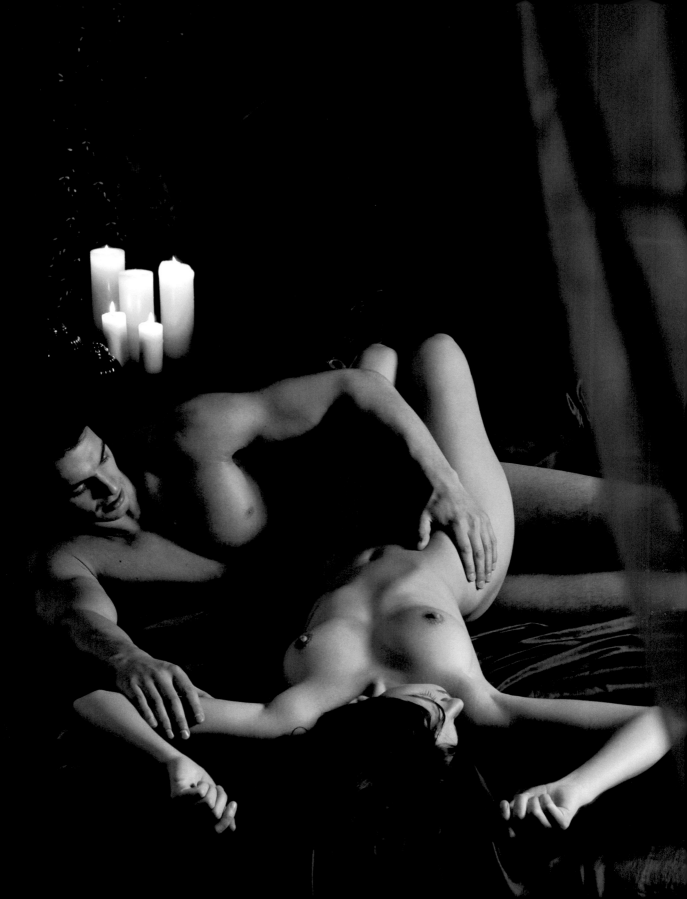

Sesamum Seed with Rice

TILATANDULAKA

*'When lovers lie on a bed, and embrace each other so closely that
the arms and thighs of the one are encircled by the arms and thighs
of the other, and are, as it were, rubbing up against them, this is called
an embrace like "the mixture of sesamum seed with rice".'*

Kama Sutra

This gentle and universally favoured position often follows on naturally from rear-entry sex once the couple have collapsed on the bed after climax, and is a perfectly natural one in which to then fall asleep. But it can also be the calm before the passion! The couple lie on their sides in a simple embrace, assuming the same foetal position as each other and in this way uniting as one. Cupping each other's bodies allows a restful closeness where intimacy can be heightened by whispering to one another or breathing in sync, whilst slowly pressing different areas of your body together. Raising her outside leg slightly, the woman squeezes the penis in the groove of her buttocks, and with very slight movements of her pelvis she simulates penetration and will delight in the feel of him hardening against her. Arching her back exposes her genitals even more so that the man can rub the tip of his penis against her labia, until she is moist and wants him inside her.

DIFFICULTY	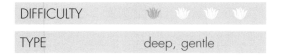
TYPE	deep, gentle

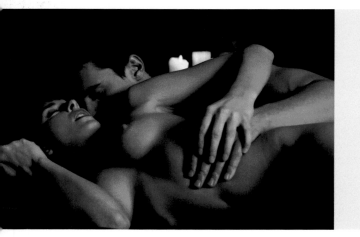

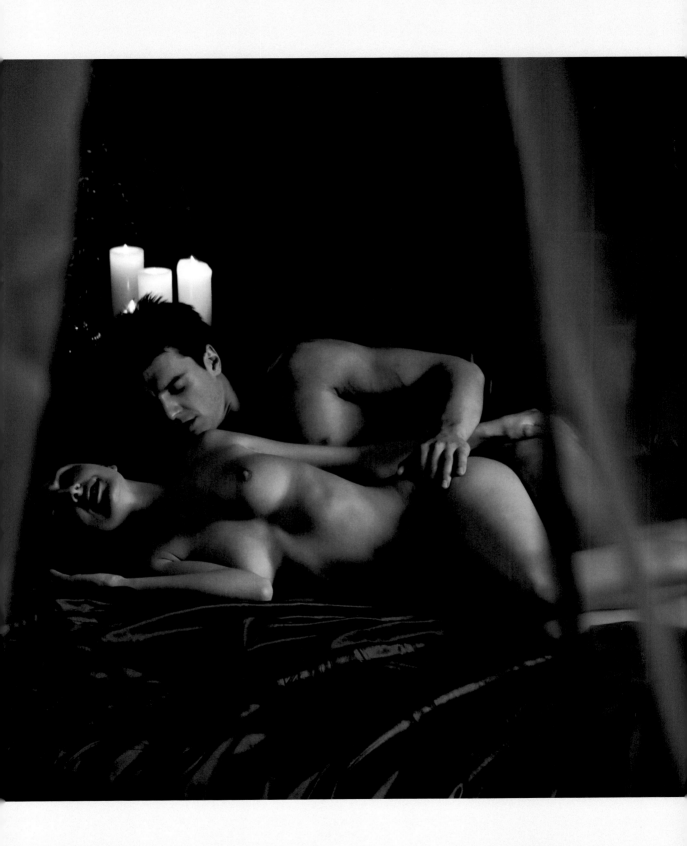

Riding the Horse

'The woman sits down, impaling herself on his member; she must not lie down, but keep seated as if on horseback, the saddle being represented by the knees and the stomach of the man. In that position she can, by the play of her knees, work up and down and down and up.'

Perfumed Garden

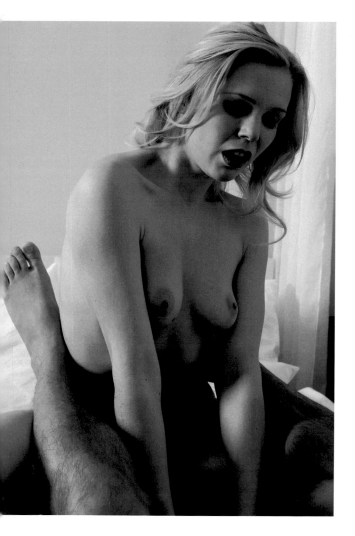

With her lover lying back comfortably, the woman kneels between his open legs. Admiring his outstretched body she can begin to touch and tease him, gently brushing her hand across his genitals as she massages his legs and abdomen.

She is in control and will find his facial expressions a big turn-on as she slowly begins to masturbate him. While he is semi-erect, the man draws his knees into his chest and his lover rises off her haunches and presses close to him so that their genitals are virtually touching.

Leaning against his thighs with his feet hooked over her shoulders she can gently push down on his penis, teasing the tip into her vagina, and once penetrated can thrust at her own desired pace.

DIFFICULTY				
TYPE	soft, slow			

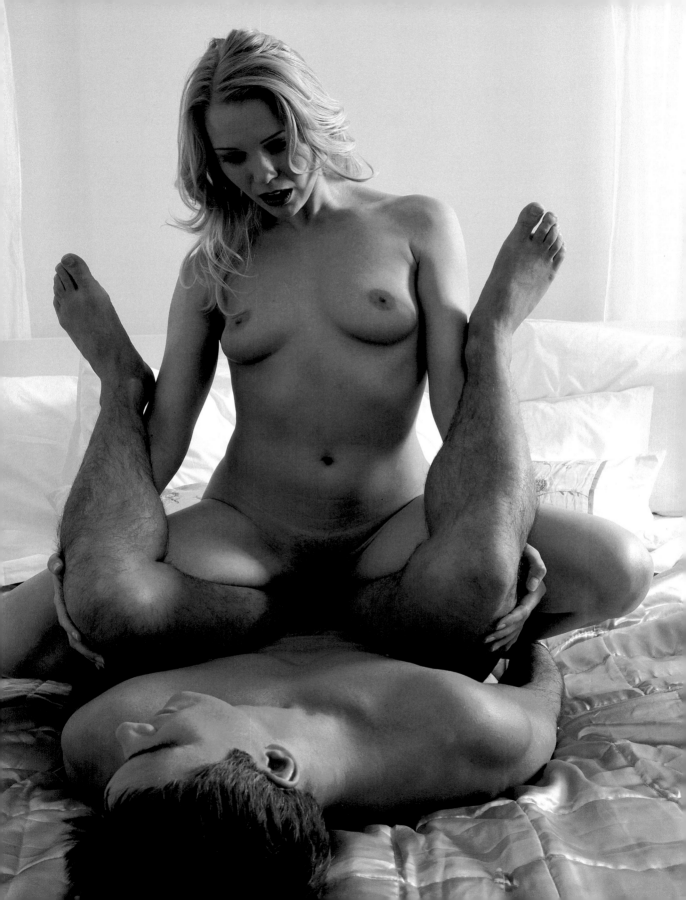

The Knot

KIRTIBANDHA

Continuing on from Riding the Horse, the woman withdraws briefly from her lover, lowers his legs and moves closer to him. She straddles his lap and wraps her legs around his waist in a loving clench. Pulling his head between her breasts, she plays with his hair and massages his scalp. For support the man can hold onto her back or prop himself against a headboard or piece of furniture, and by keeping his legs straight he provides a firmer base for her to ride him. This simple posture

is wonderful for deep, intimate penetration. Sitting higher than her lover, the woman can relish her full control as she thrusts up and down and kneads her pelvis against him whilst enjoying very close eye contact and deep, passionate kissing.

Leaning back on her arms allows her partner a good view of her outstretched chest, so that he can slowly circle his tongue around her nipples or gently nuzzle them with his nose. Because of the

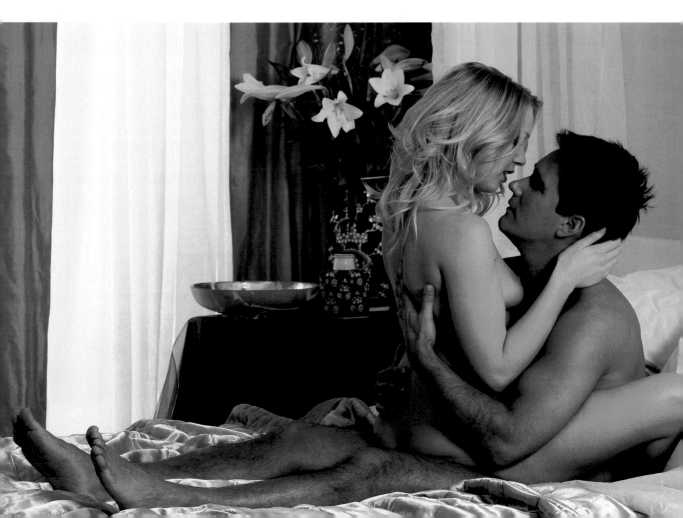

friction generated by close thrusting, this position maintains a hot bond between the lovers. It also allows the woman to sit firmly on her man so that she can enjoy the feel of his full expanse inside her.

This is a very versatile position as it can equally be used at the start of love-making, with or without penetration. It can also allow the man to get an erection, by the woman moving her hips against him while kissing him slowly and gently.

DIFFICULTY	
TYPE	deep, intense

Nakhachchhedya

Eastern erotic texts talk about marking or scratching the skin. Many people like to feel their lover's hands and nails pressing into their body, stimulating their nerve endings and making the skin tingle. The sight of scratch marks made in the heat of passion can be a great memento of your last wild encounter.

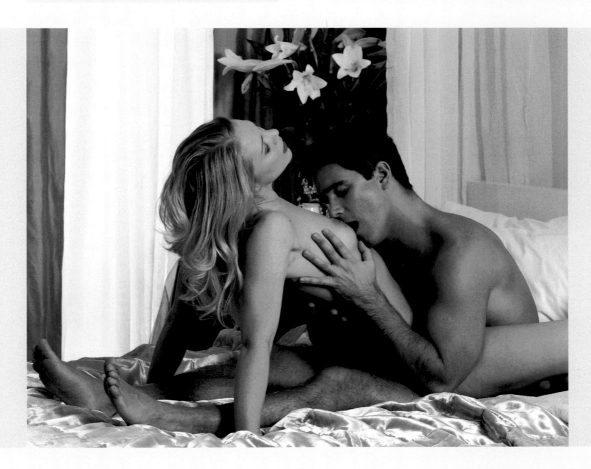

The Archimedean Screw

EL LOULABI

*'The man being stretched on his back, the woman sits on his member,
as if on a pipe through which the water of the fountain is forced,
issuing out of a narrow opening like the screw of Archimedes.'*
Perfumed Garden

This is a classic woman-on-top position. Leaning forward and taking her weight on her hands, the woman folds each of her legs so that she comes to kneel comfortably over her lover. The man reclines, giving him a full view of her astride him. If she has long hair the woman can lean forward and drape this over the man's face and chest to tickle and tantalize him. Although the man is very passive, he will take pleasure in watching her ecstatic facial expressions and seeing her breasts judder as she bounces up and down on him. Resting his head on his hands and closing his eyes, he can abandon himself to the rhythm of his lover and the sensual sound of her heavy breathing.

DIFFICULTY			
TYPE	deep, intense		

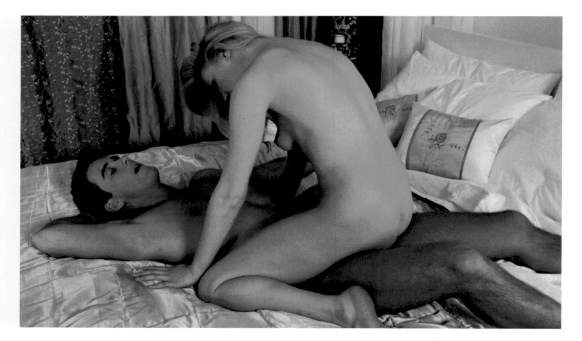

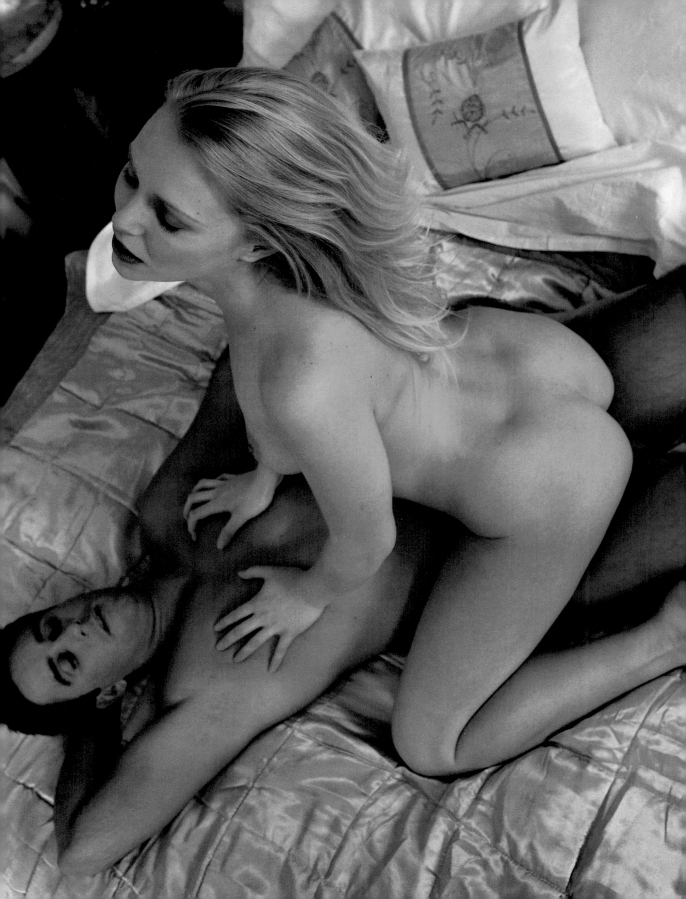

The Dominant Goddess

The woman sits upright on her man and keeps up a steady rhythm. Leaning back further increases the downward squeeze on his penis and alters the direction of penetration. The man can assist this posture by bending his legs to support the woman's buttocks, or she can place both hands on his knees to push off as she thrusts. The thrusts don't have to be vigorous to be effective, especially for the woman, as even subtle movements will give her plenty of clitoral stimulation. The man's hands are free to support her breasts throughout or, as an added stimulus, he might prefer her to fondle them and play with her nipples.

DIFFICULTY	🪷 🪷 🪷 🪷
TYPE	deep, intense

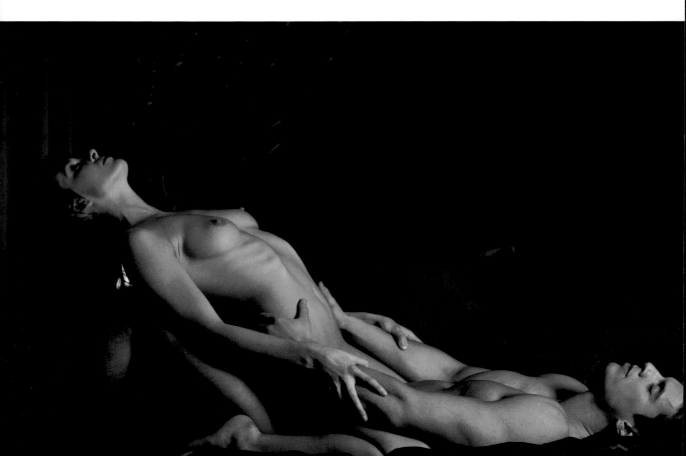

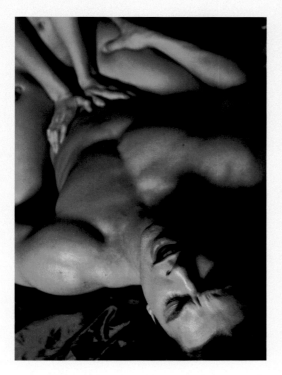

The Power of the Goddess

According to Hindu belief, every god has his corresponding goddess or consort to give him energy and strength. In the literature of India, there is often mention of goddesses on top of their gods in sexual union.

As you straddle your man, imagine that you are a life-giving, all powerful goddess and feel your sexual energy pulsing from your body into his.

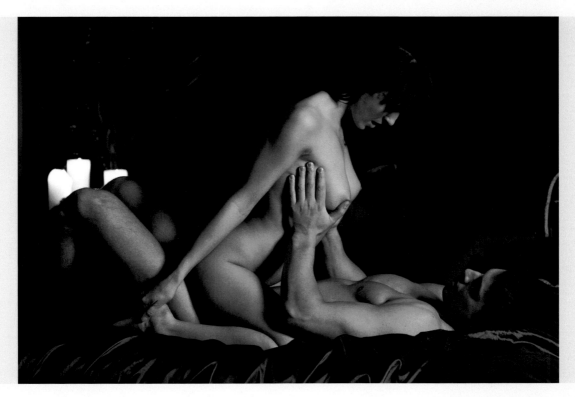

The Large Bee

'In this, the wife, having placed her husband at full length upon the bed or carpet, sits squat upon his thighs, closes her legs firmly after she has effected insertion: and, moving her waist in a circular form, churning, as it were, enjoys her husband, and thoroughly satisfies herself.'

Ananga Ranga

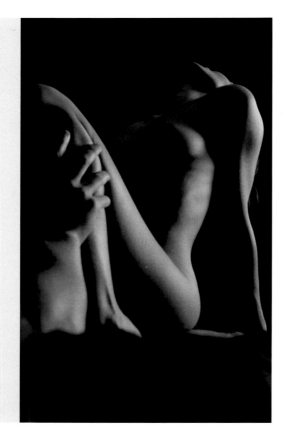

The man stretches out his legs and places his arms flat by his sides. The woman leans back and, resting her hands on his knees, she pulls up each leg and squats on his groin, being careful not to apply all her weight at once. Pressing her thighs together squeezes his penis inside her which she can vary by simply opening and closing her legs.

Any small movement in this tight pose will stimulate each partner. Swivelling her hips ensures the head of his penis hits every part of her vagina, and she can vary her strokes from side to side or forward and back. In this way, her stirring movements mimic a bee as it delves and circles for pollen inside a flower.

DIFFICULTY	
TYPE	intense, slow

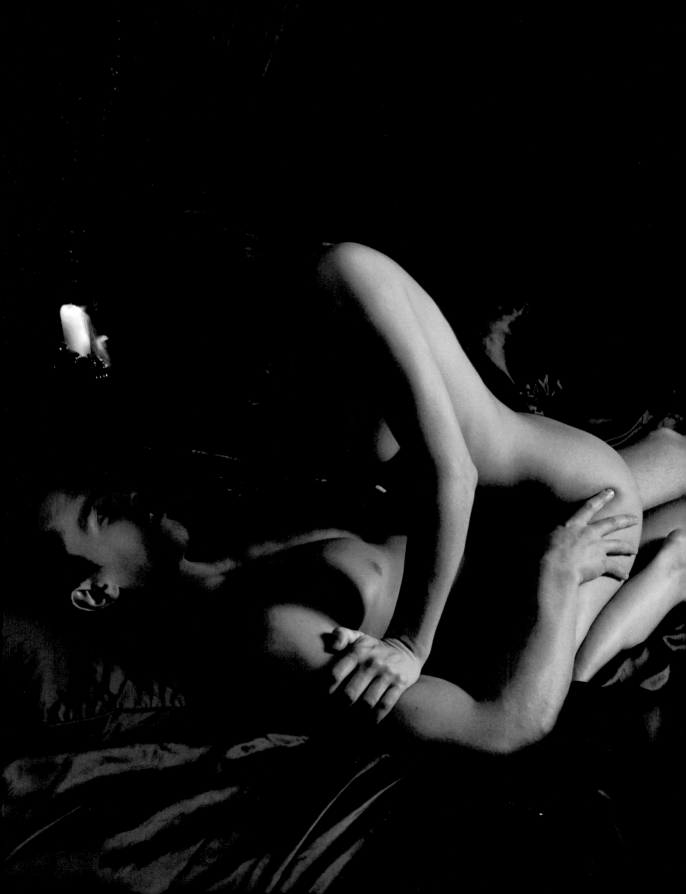

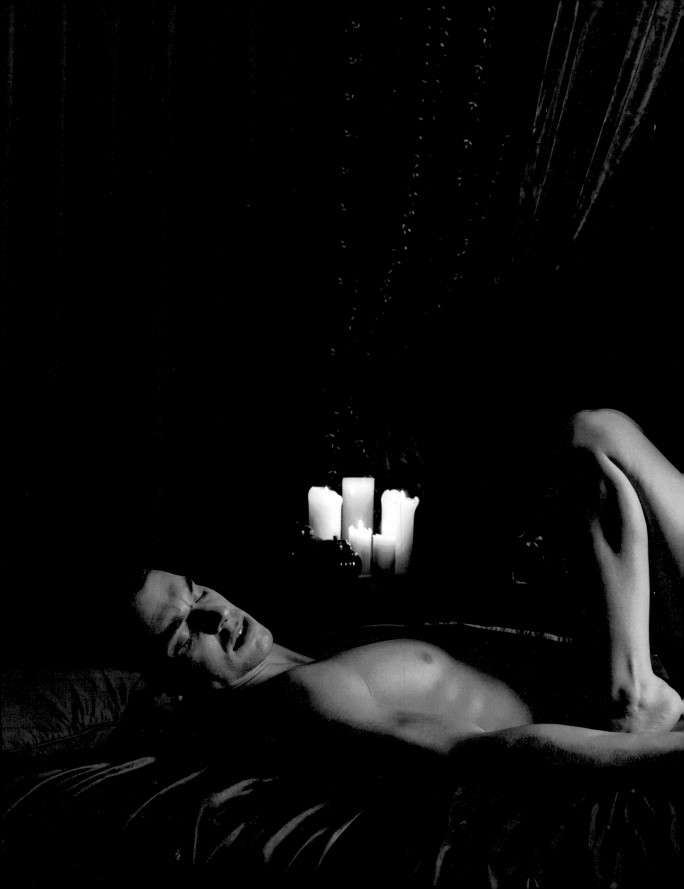

'Splendid Divalgiri, or wall lights, should gleam around the wall...whilst both man and woman should contend against any reserve, or false shame, giving themselves up in complete nakedness to unrestrained voluptuousness, upon a high and handsome bedstead...furnished with many pillows, and covered by a rich chatra, or canopy; the coverlet scented by burning luscious incense, such as aloes and other fragrant woods. In such a place, let the man, ascending the throne of love, enjoy the woman in ease and comfort, gratifying his and her every wish and every whim.'

Ananga Ranga

The Beautiful Bird

SAUMYA-BANDHA

'Saumya-Bandha is the name given by the old poets to a form of congress much in vogue amongst the artful students of the Kamashastra.'

Ananga Ranga

The couple sit facing one another with their legs apart, the woman's hooked over the man's. Caressing one another's genitals they can begin

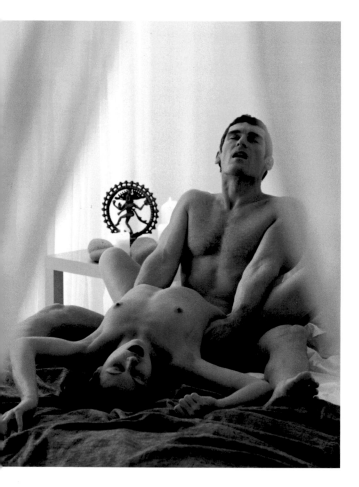

with a slow mutual masturbation, maintaining close eye contact as they do so, and leaning forward to kiss deeply now and again. Holding her hips, the man pulls his lover towards him and with her help slowly enters her. Clasping each other they can build up a good see-saw rhythm. To vary this, the woman can lean right back until she is supine, causing a sensual downward squeeze on her lover's penis and a different angle of penetration for her. The man will enjoy the view of his lover lying back and laid open, and with little strain for him in this posture he is free to explore and tease her vagina with his fingers.

She can also reach down to squeeze her labia against his penis or masturbate whilst he remains still inside her. Above all, this is a good position for experimenting with different angles and movements and an easy one for the couple to take turns pleasuring each other.

DIFFICULTY		
TYPE	deep, slow	

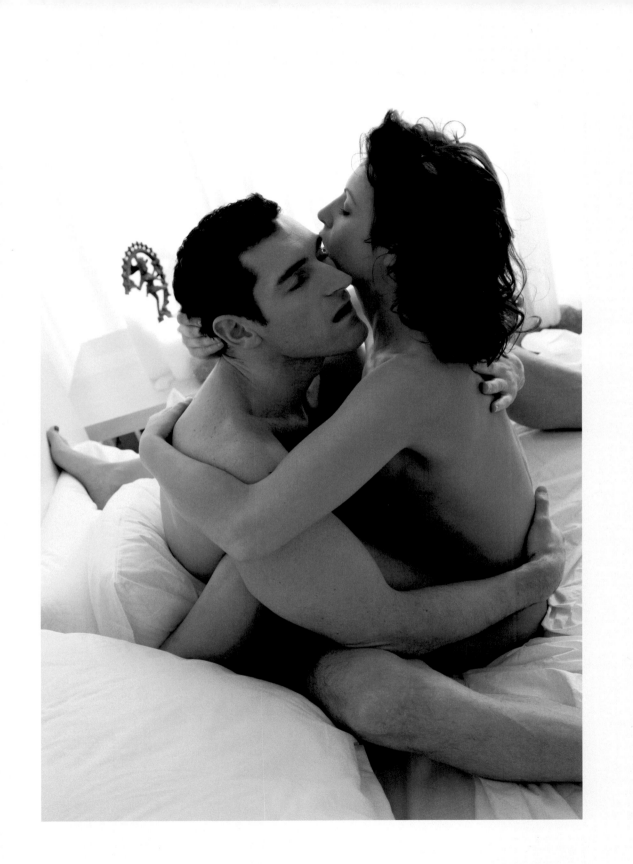

Stretching the Legs

'The husband places the wife upon her back, raises both her legs and, placing them upon his shoulders, sits close to her and enjoys her.'

Ananga Ranga

Once the couple has enjoyed the slow build-up of sexual tension in The Beautiful Bird, the woman opens herself out like a blossoming flower and extends her legs onto the man's shoulders, giving him an unfettered view of her bud. Being thus outstretched allows her sexual energies to flow more powerfully through her body.

For the man, seeing his lover's yoni displayed invitingly before him gives an added turn-on that will help maintain his erection. The man places his legs either side of her body and then penetrates her. He will find that watching the movement of her breasts as he moves in and out of her, as well as her facial expressions of pleasure and desire adds to his arousal.

In this position, the man may need to lean against a sofa or a headboard for back support, and this posture will be easier for those with supple legs and strong pelvic muscle control. He can pull her hips towards him to allow deeper penetration or withdraw from her. Gently stroking her labia and rubbing her clitoris will keep them both fully aroused if they want to continue penetration.

Alternatively, he may just tease her with the tip of his penis before resuming coition. The depth of penetration in this position can combine passion with intimacy beautifully.

DIFFICULTY	🌸 🌸 ⚪ ⚪
TYPE	deep, gentle, slow

Pelvic Floor Exercises

These can be done anywhere because nobody can tell you are doing them. Squeeze the muscles, as if you are trying to stop the flow of urine (the best way to understand what this means is to try stopping the flow of urine when you are actually on the toilet). Try pulsing the muscles both slowly and quickly. Place one or two fingers inside your vagina so you can find out how this would feel on your man. If you do this exercise daily, the muscles will soon become so strong that you will be able to keep hold of even the strongest stallion!

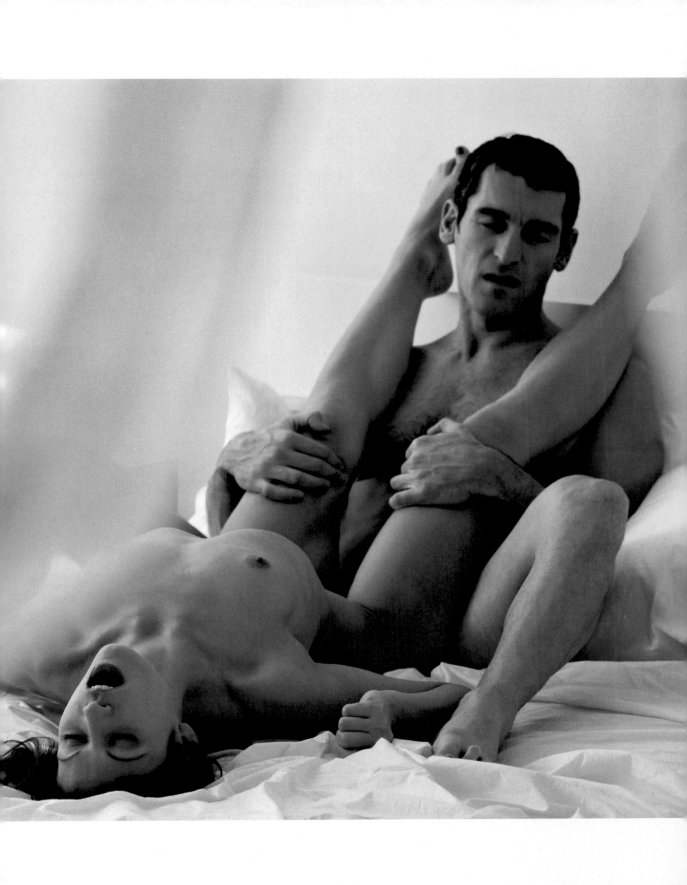

The Crab

KARKATA

'There takes place between the two actors wrestling, intertwinings, a kind of animated conflict... The man is at work as with a pestle, while the woman seconds him by lascivious movements; finally comes the ejaculation.'
Perfumed Garden

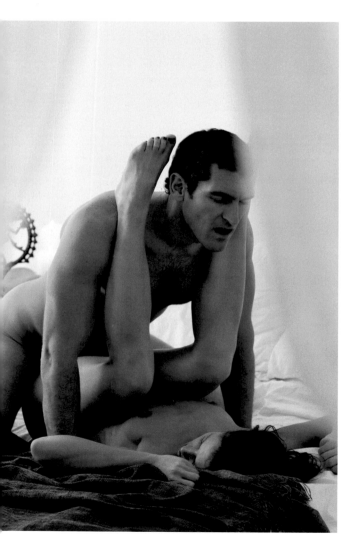

This is a lusty position to get into once lovers are so filled with carnal desire that they need a quick and urgent release. Lifting the woman's legs in front of him and holding them together, the man rises into a kneeling position. The woman draws her knees towards her chest, which shortens and tightens her vagina, so that even shallow thrusts will press all the right buttons.

She could raise her buttocks up on cushions to allow a deeper sensation for the man. He leans over her, dominant and in control. From this position, he could surprise her by withdrawing suddenly and moving his mouth to her clitoris, sucking and licking it vigorously before resuming penetration.

As they near climax, the man and woman can gaze into each other's eyes, acknowledging the intense experience they have just shared.

DIFFICULTY	🌸 🌸 🌸
TYPE	deep, intense, fast

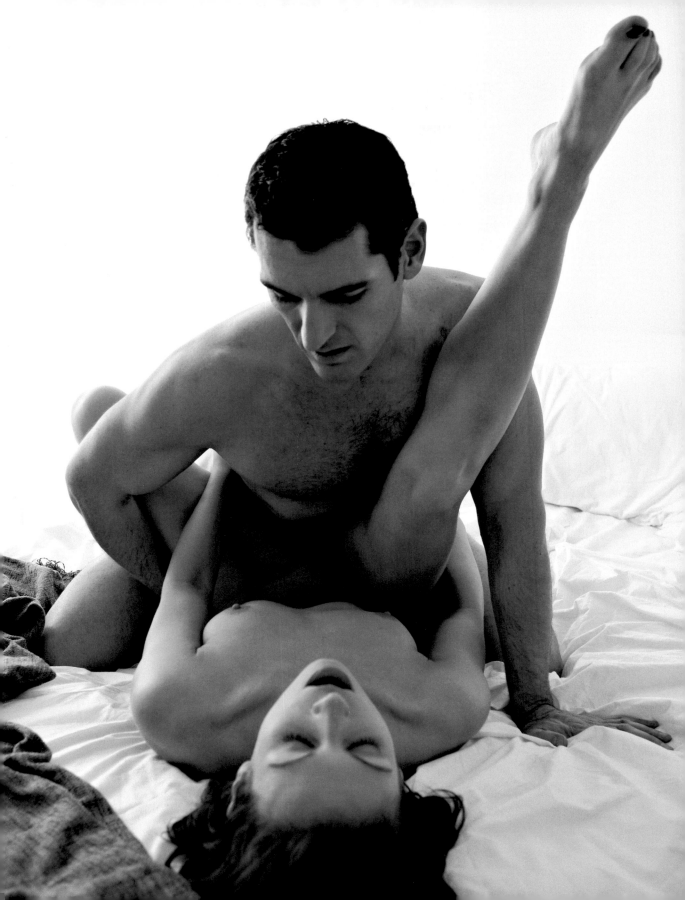

The Congress of a Herd of Cows

GAUYUTHIKA

'When a man enjoys many women altogether, it is called the Gauyuthika or "the congress of a herd of cows"...Just as it is possible for a man to unite with two or more women at the same time, so it is possible for the woman to unite with two or more men at the same time. When one woman unites with two men, it is named Sanghataka or "the united congress". When she unites with many men, it is called Gauyuthika or "the congress of a herd of cows".'

The ancient temples and paintings of India often depict group sex sessions. It is a timeless sexual pursuit – many men and women today like to indulge in wild orgies, partner swapping and swinging. If you are open and confident with your lover, this can add another exciting dimension to your sex life.

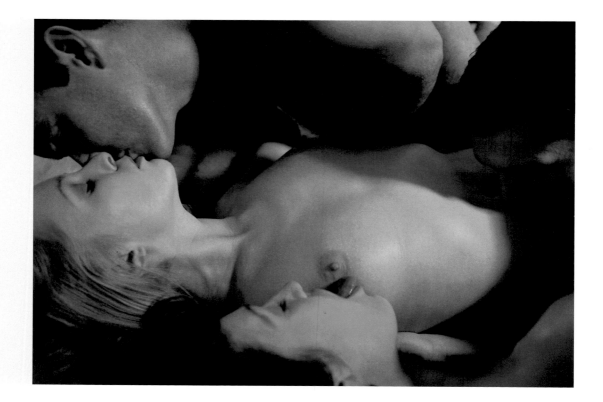

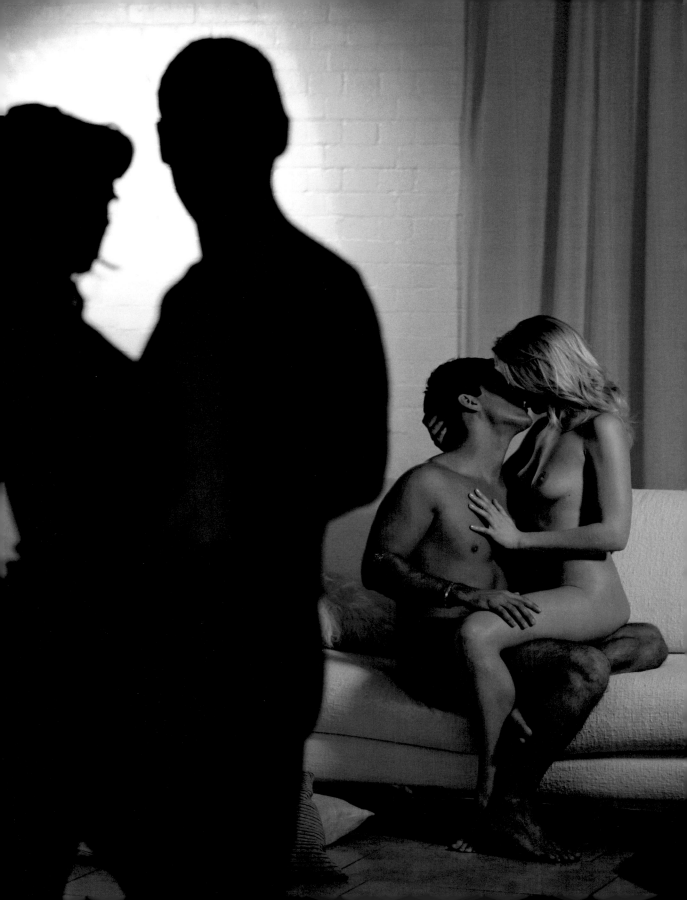

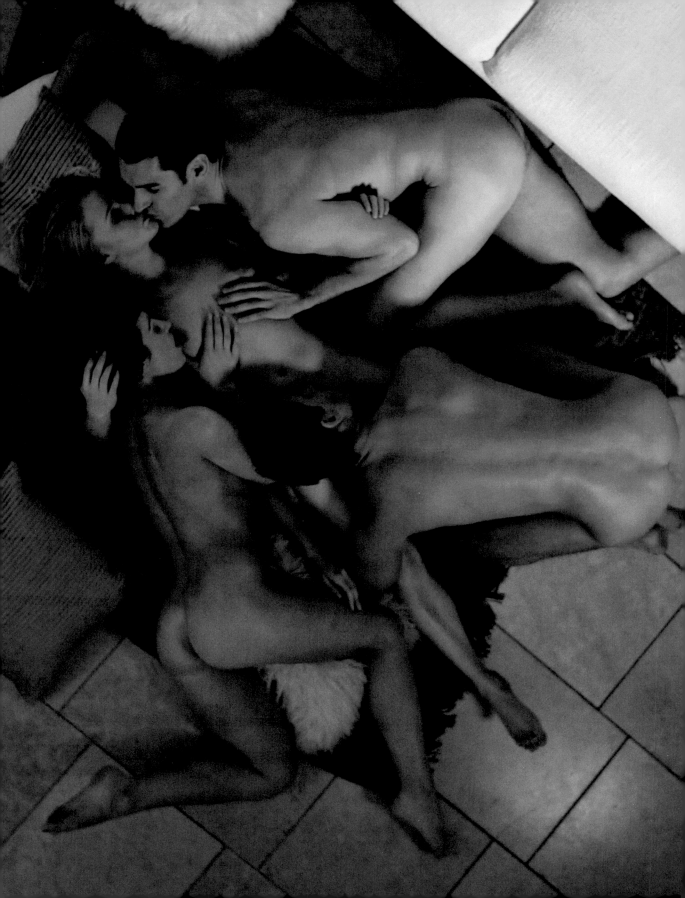

'In the provinces of Gramaneri
many young men enjoy a woman
that may be married to one of them,
either one after the other or at the
same time. Thus one young man
holds her, another unites with her,
a third uses her mouth, a fourth
holds her middle part, and in this
way they go on enjoying her
several parts alternately.'

Kama Sutra

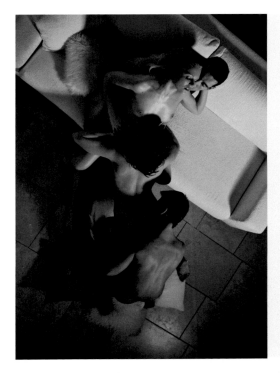

'The same things can be done when
several men are sitting in company
with one courtesan, or when one
courtesan is alone with many men.'

Kama Sutra

INDEX